Living with Multiple Sclerosis

Mark Greener spent a decade in biomedical research before joining *MIMS Magazine* for GPs in 1989. Since then, he has written on health and biology for magazines worldwide for patients, healthcare professionals and scientists. He is a member of the Royal Society of Biology and clinical editor for *Pharmacy Magazine*. He is the author of 24 other books, including *The Heart Attack Survival Guide* (2012), *The Holistic Health Handbook* (2013) and *The Holistic Guide for Cancer Survivors* (2016), all published by Sheldon Press.

Overcoming Common Problems Series

Selected titles

A full list of titles is available from Sheldon Press,
36 Causton Street, London SW1P 4ST and on our website at
www.sheldonpress.co.uk

Beating Insomnia: Without really trying
Dr Tim Cantopher

Birth Over 35
Sheila Kitzinger

Breast Cancer: Your treatment choices
Dr Terry Priestman

Chronic Fatigue Syndrome: What you need to know about CFS/ME
Dr Megan A. Arroll

The Chronic Pain Diet Book
Neville Shone

Cider Vinegar
Margaret Hills

Coeliac Disease: What you need to know
Alex Gazzola

Coping Successfully with Chronic Illness: Your healing plan
Neville Shone

Coping Successfully with Hiatus Hernia
Dr Tom Smith

Coping Successfully with Pain
Neville Shone

Coping Successfully with Panic Attacks
Shirley Trickett

Coping Successfully with Prostate Cancer
Dr Tom Smith

Coping Successfully with Shyness
Margaret Oakes, Professor Robert Bor and Dr Carina Eriksen

Coping Successfully with Ulcerative Colitis
Peter Cartwright

Coping Successfully with Varicose Veins
Christine Craggs-Hinton

Coping Successfully with Your Irritable Bowel
Rosemary Nicol

Coping with a Mental Health Crisis: Seven steps to healing
Catherine G. Lucas

Coping with Anaemia
Dr Tom Smith

Coping with Asthma in Adults
Mark Greener

Coping with Blushing
Professor Robert J. Edelmann

Coping with Bronchitis and Emphysema
Dr Tom Smith

Coping with Chemotherapy
Dr Terry Priestman

Coping with Coeliac Disease: Strategies to change your diet and life
Karen Brody

Coping with Difficult Families
Dr Jane McGregor and Tim McGregor

Coping with Diverticulitis
Peter Cartwright

Coping with Dyspraxia
Jill Eckersley

Coping with Early-onset Dementia
Jill Eckersley

Coping with Endometriosis
Jill Eckersley and Dr Zara Aziz

Coping with Envy: Feeling at a disadvantage with friends and family
Dr Windy Dryden

Coping with Epilepsy
Dr Pamela Crawford and Fiona Marshall

Coping with Gout
Christine Craggs-Hinton

Coping with Guilt
Dr Windy Dryden

Coping with Headaches and Migraine
Alison Frith

Coping with Heartburn and Reflux
Dr Tom Smith

Coping with Life after Stroke
Dr Mareeni Raymond

Coping with Liver Disease
Mark Greener

Coping with Memory Problems
Dr Sallie Baxendale

Coping with Obsessive Compulsive Disorder
Professor Kevin Gournay, Rachel Piper and Professor Paul Rogers

Coping with Pet Loss
Robin Grey

Coping with Phobias and Panic
Professor Kevin Gournay

Overcoming Common Problems Series

Overcoming Common Problems Series

Overcoming Common Problems

Living with Multiple Sclerosis

MARK GREENER

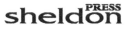

First published in Great Britain in 2017

Sheldon Press
36 Causton Street
London SW1P 4ST
www.sheldonpress.co.uk

The author and publisher have made every effort to ensure that the
external website and email addresses included in this book are correct and
up to date at the time of going to press. The author and publisher are not
responsible for the content, quality or continuing accessibility of the sites.

British Library Cataloguing-in-Publication Data
A catalogue record for this book is available from the British Library

ISBN 978-1-84709-413-1
eBook ISBN 978-1-84709-414-8

Typeset by Fakenham Prepress Solutions, Fakenham, Norfolk NR21 8NN
First printed in Great Britain by Ashford Colour Press
Subsequently digitally reprinted in Great Britain

eBook by Fakenham Prepress Solutions, Fakenham, Norfolk NR21 8NN

Produced on paper from sustainable forests

To Rose, Yasmin, Rory and Ophelia for their love and support

Contents

Note to the reader

This is not a medical book and is not intended to replace advice from your doctor. Consult your pharmacist, MS team or doctor if you believe you have any of the symptoms described, and if you think you might need medical help.

Introduction

Your brain is easily the most remarkable organ in your body. After all, the brain is, the American writer Ambrose Bierce quipped, the 'apparatus with which we think that we think'. This soft blob – writers compare its consistency to a jelly, soft tofu or warm butter – is responsible for your intelligence, emotions and personality. And the brain is connected to a network of nerves that control your movements, interpret the world around you and allow you to perform the activities of everyday life. We take the brain and nervous system for granted – until something goes wrong.

Nerves connect your brain to every part of your body, from the hair follicles in your scalp, to the end of your big toe, to your fingertips. This network of nerves means that you immediately know when someone pulls your hair, you stub your toe or you touch a hot pan. In turn, the brain passes signals along the nerves to the organs that keep us alive: our lungs, heart and gut, for example. These signalling pathways ensure that your body adapts to meet your changing needs, whether you are walking to the shops, reading this book or playing with your children.

Multiple sclerosis (MS) arises when your body attacks some of these nerve pathways. The interruptions to the nerve signals results in the difficulties faced by people with MS – such as issues with walking, unpleasant sensations and poor balance – that all too often take their toll on you physically, mentally and emotionally.

A sneaky disease

Often MS seems to 'sneak up' on the person. The first signs may be barely noticeable: a little dizziness, some 'pins and needles', taking longer to complete a routine task or making more mistakes at work.[1, 2] Some people lose their ability to perform fine actions, such as texting. These kinds of difficulties can have a variety of causes, including other diseases, age and being 'just one of those things' that passes. Even so, in the UK, about one person every two hours receives the distressing news that he or she has MS.

In other words, MS is relatively common. The MS Society estimates that about 1 person in every 600 in the UK lives with MS. Yet MS remains poorly understood, enigmatic and incurable.

Despite extensive research, we still do not really understand what causes MS. We do not really understand why the signs, symptoms and course differ so widely from person to person: 1 in 10 people with MS does not experience a progressive decline that ends in disability, but some rare forms can rapidly kill. Also, we do not fully understand why MS seems to be becoming more common. It is likely, however, that changes in lifestyle and environment are involved. As we'll see, researchers link several risk factors with MS, including certain viruses, cigarette smoking, a lack of vitamin D (the 'sunshine' vitamin), what we eat (our diet) and the genes we inherit from our biological parents. For instance, MS is about 10 times more common among white people living in the UK than in South Africa. Genes contribute to the differences in MS risk around the world. However, the environment – especially certain infections and vitamin D – is also influential.[3] Environmental differences seem to be why rates of MS are lower than expected in Northern Norway, Japan and Alaska.[4] We'll look at what these differences mean to people in the UK.

An incurable disease

A cure for MS remains a distant prospect. Nevertheless, a growing number of drugs can transform the prospects for many – but sadly not all – people with MS. These drugs (and many more are being developed) can modify the course of some forms of MS, reducing the number of times when symptoms worsen or new difficulties arise ('relapses') and, in some cases, delaying disability. They do not, however, totally prevent relapses. These 'disease-modifying drugs' dramatically improve the quality of life for some people with MS. Occasionally, however, these drugs cause serious side effects.

Despite therapeutic advances, it is easy to feel overwhelmed, disempowered, frightened and depressed when you face MS. After all, your immune system, which usually protects you from infections, seems to have turned against you. In most people with MS, the attack by the immune system slowly destroys the nerves. So, on average, a person with MS develops 'significant disability' eight years after diagnosis.[5] You may feel you can do little to improve your prospects. If this book has one message, it is that this is not true.

Indeed, conventional MS management draws on the expertise of several groups of health professionals to help you live as full a life as possible. In addition to a doctor who is an expert in diseases of the nervous system (neurologist), you may be treated by a dietitian, physiotherapist, pharmacist or occupational therapist. In many hospitals, a nurse who specializes in MS might coordinate your care and be your first port of call if you have issues or questions. Increasingly, these nurses have an additional qualification that allows them to prescribe certain medicines. This 'multidisciplinary' approach allows the MS team to develop an individualized programme that meets your changing needs. You can build on the foundation provided by your MS teams using complementary and alternative medicines (CAM), a variety of self-help techniques and lifestyle changes.

In the prime of life

MS often strikes people who are in the prime of their lives: 6 in every 7 people with MS were younger than 50 years of age when they were diagnosed.[6] (We will focus in this book on adults, as MS is rare in childhood.[3]) Indeed, other than injury, MS is the most common cause of chronic (long-lasting) disability among young adults in the UK.[7]

The effects of MS are often more than physical. Not surprisingly, depression and anxiety are more common among people with MS than the population as a whole. The depression and anxiety are partly reactions to the stress of living with a serious, unpredictable, potentially disabling disease. In addition, depression and anxiety may follow damage to parts of the brain that control emotions. MS can also undermine cognitive (your intellect and memory) performance. This, in turn, can compromise, for instance, your independence, employment, social and recreational activities and driving skills.[8] These difficulties can wax and wane as you, for example, recover from a relapse or come to terms with MS.

Nevertheless, the physical and mental changes can mean that MS can alter, and sometimes strain, family relationships. A person with

MS may need to change careers or leave work. A wife who was the main carer for her family while working may need care and only be able to work part time. Sadly, the divorce rate is twice that of the rest of the population when one partner has MS.[3]

Understanding MS helps you limit, as far as possible, the stress and impact on your relationships. That is one of the reasons many people with MS turn to CAMs. *These never replace conventional therapies.* Nevertheless, many people with MS find that CAMs improve their quality of life and may help alleviate, for example, pain, fatigue and psychological symptoms. CAMs can also help people feel more in control of their lives and disease, rather than that their MS controls them.

Enigmatic, capricious and unpredictable

The bravery that most people show when they face MS never ceases to amaze and inspire me. Nevertheless, your MS journey is deeply personal, often difficult and at times frightening for you and your family. Although, for example, disability usually takes many years to develop, it casts a long shadow. I hope that the suggestions in this book will make life a little easier for you and your family.

MS is, however, enigmatic, capricious and unpredictable. Despite scans that can now image your brain and spinal cord in remarkable detail, no one can precisely predict how the disease might progress. Even people with the same 'type' of MS show widely different trajectories. Likewise, no one can accurately predict how well the treatments will work for you. Your MS team offers educated guesses based on scientific data gained from many thousands of people, but countless people with MS have defied their doctor's expectations.

No one can guarantee that the suggestions in the book will definitely work for you. If you feel that any of them might help, always check with your MS team. The aim of the suggestions and information is to support the treatment from your MS team – they are not replacements. The advice from your MS team is tailored to your particular situation, goals and circumstances, and overrides the suggestions in this book. Always contact your GP or MS team if you feel unwell or think that your disease is getting worse, even if it is between appointments. As Roger McDougall, a Scottish scriptwriter and playwright who developed MS, commented, 'there is no one and only way to control multiple sclerosis . . . no one and only cause, no one and only way to help even one individual'.[1]

A note about references

It is impossible to cite all the numerous medical and scientific studies that I used to write this book (apologies to anyone whose work I missed). I have highlighted certain papers to illustrate important points and themes. You can find a summary of these papers by entering the details here: <www.ncbi.nlm.nih.gov/pubmed>. Some full-length papers are available online free or at a reduced rate for patients. Larger libraries may stock or allow you to access some medical journals. Some of the papers may seem rather erudite if you do not have a medical or biological background, but do not let that put you off. If you feel you do not understand something, please ask your GP, pharmacist, MS team or a helpline run by a charity.

1

What is MS?

With the benefit of hindsight, healers seemed to have first recognized the cluster of symptoms we now call MS during the fourteenth century. Nevertheless, it was not until 1868 that the great French neurologist Jean-Martin Charcot linked the signs of MS with characteristic scarring (page 8) in the brain and spinal cord.[9] Yet, despite almost 150 years of intensive research, MS remains, in the words of one medical textbook, 'a disease of paradoxes and questions'.[6]

A common condition

It's clear, however, that MS is common. According to the MS Society, about 107,000 people live with MS in the UK. Another 5000 people are diagnosed with MS each year – about one person every two hours. Also, MS is becoming more common. A study from Norway, for example, found that the number of people living with MS increased tenfold between 1963 and 2013.[10] Likewise, a UK study suggested that the number of people with MS increased by about 1 in 40 (2.4 per cent) steadily year after year between 1990 and 2010.[5]

Several factors probably drive the increase in number of people living with MS. For example, doctors diagnose MS more quickly today than in the past. That is partly a reflection of there being greater awareness of MS among doctors and the public and partly a result of technological innovation. Since the 1990s, for example, neurologists have used magnetic resonance imaging (MRI; page 37) to identify the hallmarks of MS in the brain and spinal cord. The brain scans mean neurologists no longer have to rely on physical signs (such as measuring changes in the speed at which the nerve signal travels) and symptoms (pain and movement difficulties, for example), both of which can be misleading.

As we will see, neurologists do not diagnose MS until they are sure you have the disease (Chapter 3). Brain scans do often reveal subtle early stages, however, and mean that neurologists tend to diagnose MS in younger people than in the past. These scans also mean that doctors can detect less serious, and more symptomatically ambiguous, cases of MS.[5] Some of these cases, especially if mild, probably used to slip under the doctors' radar in the past until movement difficulties and other symptoms emerged.

Finally, environmental and behavioural changes also seem to contribute to the increase in MS.[10] There is now little doubt, for example, that sunlight protects against MS, almost certainly by producing vitamin D (page 24).[3] We spend less time outdoors than in the past and, when we venture out, tend to use high-factor sunscreen. Applying sun protection factor (SPF) 8 and SPF 15 sunscreens can reduce the amount of vitamin D produced by 92.5 per cent and 99 per cent respectively.[11] (You do not need much sunlight to get enough vitamin D – see page 25 – so the risk of MS is not a reason to ditch the sunblock.)

Mortality in MS

Typically, people tend to die *with* rather than *from* MS. In 2010, overall life expectancy was about 78 (78.3) years in men and almost 82 (81.8) years in women. In people with MS, life expectancy was about 65 (65.4) years in men and almost 72 (71.6) years in women.[5] However, rare and aggressive forms of MS can directly cause death. Moreover, the disability that is often associated with MS can make other diseases more common, including some infections, mental health symptoms, diabetes and heart conditions.

The movement difficulties experienced by some people with MS can make exercise difficult and lack of exercise can contribute to anxiety, diabetes and heart disease. Largely because of these issues, a person with MS has a life expectancy about ten years shorter than that of the general population. Logically, if drugs can reduce the number of relapses and delay or prevent disability, they will help keep people active, so the average lifespan of people with MS may be increasing. Many newer drugs have not been around long enough to see if they improve lifespan and by how much.[3]

More common in women and white people

Some people are especially likely to develop MS. For example, about 7 in every 10 cases of MS in the UK occur in women.[5] However, the size of this difference depends on the person's age. In children, three girls may develop MS for every boy. Among people in their forties, however, roughly similar numbers of men and women develop MS. Genetic studies have not found any link to the X and Y chromosomes that determine sex, so the reason for the difference is not clear.[6]

MS also seems to be more common among white people than those from black and South Asian ethnic backgrounds. A study from east London, for example, reported that people of black and South Asian origin were three-fifths and four-fifths (59 per cent and 84 per cent), respectively, less likely to develop MS than white people.[7] Studies from the other side of the Atlantic suggest that, after allowing for other risk factors, African-American men are about two-fifths (40 per cent) less likely to develop MS than their white counterparts.[6]

Differences in your skin colour are obviously related to your ancestors' exposure to sunlight. Increased skin pigmentation can reduce vitamin D production by up to 99 per cent.[11] However, in parts of the world where dark skin evolved, the intense sunlight ensured that people produced enough of this essential vitamin. Clearly, the sun is a lot weaker in the West Midlands than the West Indies. That might help explain why the risk of developing MS seems to be 'several times' higher among people of black and South Asian origin in the UK than among those living in sub-Saharan Africa or South Asia. The difference probably also reflects the greater likelihood of being diagnosed with MS in the relatively affluent UK than in countries with more impoverished health services.[7]

Your nerves

So what do we know about what goes wrong in people with MS? We need to begin by looking at a healthy nervous system.

Nerves are the 'wires' that carry tiny electrical signals around your body. When you need to turn the page of this book, nerves carry the signal from your brain to your fingers. Pinch yourself gently.

Nerves carry a signal from the pinched skin to your brain. Nerves from your eye carry the image of this 'word' to your brain, which interprets the information. So, hopefully, you can understand what you are reading. Nerves spread signals from your senses around the different parts of the brain that 'need to know'. This allows you to respond to your environment.

Two broad systems

Nerves vary in diameter from 1 to 20 micrometres[12] – a micrometre being a millionth of a meter. A standard sheet of paper is about 100 micrometres thick, so you could fit between 5 and 100 nerves across the thickness of a piece of paper.

Biologists divide nerves into two broad systems.

- The **central nervous system (CNS)** consists of the brain and spinal cord. Damage to the CNS caused by MS can affect, for example, intellectual abilities, undermine memory or result in abnormal and inappropriate expressions of emotion (one woman with MS laughed during a funeral). Tingling sensations and changes in sensitivity to heat are, for instance, common in MS and seem to follow damage to the CNS pathways that carry information from the skin, joints and muscles along the spinal cord and into the brain.[13]
- The **peripheral nervous system** carries messages to and from the brain and spinal cord. Most nerves from the peripheral nervous system feed into or arise from your spinal cord and, in turn, run to and from your brain. The longest nerves run for an average of a metre from the base of the spine to the toes.[14] However, nerves feeding the head and eyes do not go through the spinal cord. As we will see, MS damages the CNS, but spares the peripheral nervous system.

Biologists further divide the peripheral nervous system into two parts.

- The **'somatic' or 'voluntary' nervous system** allows us to choose an action. Your voluntary nervous system tells your muscles to turn the pages of a book.
- The **'autonomic' or 'involuntary' nervous system** maintains our body's essential functions – such as digestion, breathing and heartbeat – without conscious control. You're doing all these as

you're reading: you don't need to think about breaking down your lunch, breathing or pumping blood around your body.

Poor control exerted by the CNS over the peripheral nervous system can cause difficulty for people living with MS. Thus, damage to the CNS may mean that the voluntary nervous system no longer receives the signals it needs to meet your demands.

A complex system

It is difficult to grasp just how complex our nervous system is. The human brain probably contains around 86 billion nerve cells.[15] That's 12 nerve cells for every man, woman and child on Earth. If you laid all your nerve cells end to end, they would measure 150,000 to 180,000 km. In other words, the nerve cells in your brain could go around the equator four times.

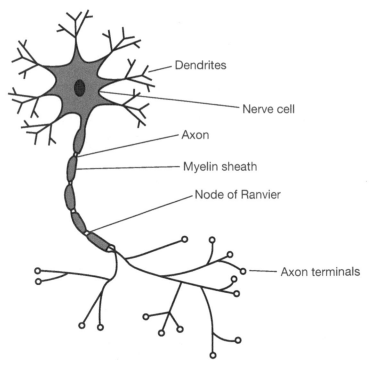

Figure 1 A typical nerve cell

Each nerve cell has numerous 'arms', called dendrites (Figure 1). Some nerve cells have thousands of dendrites. These receive signals from other nerve cells. When the total input crosses a threshold, a pulse of electrical activity travels along the nerve.

This pulse of activity usually triggers the release of chemical messengers (called neurotransmitters) from the axon terminal that pass the signal to the next nerve in the pathway or tell a muscle to contract or relax. This integrated system allows us to make the finely tuned responses we need for movement, thought, memory and the basic functions that keep us alive.[15] Incidentally, many drugs used to treat MS and other ailments work by blocking or mimicking these chemical messengers.

The developing brain

An adult's brain weighs about 1.3 to 1.4 kg (3 pounds). The brain of a newborn baby weighs about a third that of his or her parents. Within a year, the baby's brain is about three-quarters of its adult size. Babies are born with almost the same number of nerve cells as adults, but babies have far fewer connections between nerves. A newborn baby's brain makes 40,000 connections per second. This accounts for most of the rapid increase in brain size in the first year of life.[15] Clearly, anything that disrupts this rapid development could be detrimental in later life. As we will see, some risk factors for MS seem to act early in life to influence the developing brain. This seems to manifest as the physical symptoms of MS in later life.

Rapid travel

Nerve signals need to travel rapidly to meet your needs and ensure you prevent as much damage as possible. You need to increase your heartbeat, breathing and endurance rapidly when you suddenly realize you're about to miss your train, for instance. You need to know almost immediately when you touch a hot pan to get your hand out of harm's way.

Introducing myelin

A fatty layer that covers and protects many nerves – the myelin sheath (Figure 1) – is essential for the rapid flow of much of the information along the nerves that run to and from your brain. If you cut a brain or spinal cord in half, you can see two areas: the grey matter and the white matter. Areas dense in neurones look grey – literally your grey matter. Myelin gives the white matter its characteristic colour, but there's also some myelin in the grey matter.[3]

The myelin sheath is a bit like the insulation that surrounds an electrical wire. However, the myelin sheath contains regular gaps – almost as if the insulation on a wire has been rubbed away, exposing the copper beneath. These gaps are the 'nodes of Ranvier', named after the French researcher who first noticed the intervals (Figure 1). The nerve signal jumps between the nodes.

Jumping between the nodes of Ranvier allows nerve signals to travel very rapidly.[12] An unmyelinated nerve transmits signals at 0.6 to 2 metres a second – that's about walking pace (1 to 5 miles per hour). A large myelinated nerve, such as one transmitting signals telling your muscles to move, transmits signals at 60 to 120 metres a second – that's about 130 to 270 miles an hour,[12] which is faster than the top speed of a Formula 1 car. Not surprisingly, losing myelin can dramatically undermine how well your nerves work.

Other essential cells

In addition to nerves, the CNS contains numerous other essential cells.

- **Oligodendrocytes** form the myelin sheath. Several tentacle-like 'processes' reach out from the oligodendrocytes and wrap around an axon. These processes encircle the nerves in layers of myelin. The gap between adjacent oligodendrocytes creates the nodes of Ranvier. Each oligodendrocyte can send processes to up to 60 nerves.[12]
- **Microglia** respond to signals released by oligodendrocytes and other cells and are important in the brain's inflammatory responses.[16] Inflammation is an important weapon in our immune defences: it helps fight infection and encourages healing.[16] However, uncontrolled inflammation contributes to several diseases, including MS.
- **Star-shaped astrocytes** support and nourish nerves. Astrocytes

also form a scaffold that helps guide nerve cells during development and fine-tune levels of neurotransmitters in the CNS.[17]

MS can also damage these other cells.[3] Indeed, healthy nerves may no longer work properly if these cells and the supporting environment become damaged.[6]

Guillain–Barré syndrome

Like MS, Guillain–Barré syndrome follows the loss of myelin (demyelination) around nerves, but Guillain–Barré syndrome affects the peripheral nervous system rather than the CNS. As a result, people with Guillain–Barré syndrome may notice weakness or tingling sensations in their legs, often on both sides of the body. The sensation may spread to the person's arms and upper body. In severe cases, the person may have difficulties with breathing, blood pressure or heart rate, or become paralysed.

Typically, Guillain–Barré syndrome develops after an abnormal immune reaction to an infection or inflammation, so may emerge a few days or weeks after a respiratory (lung) or gastrointestinal viral infection. Occasionally surgery and, in very rare cases, vaccinations may trigger Guillain–Barré syndrome. Most people make a good recovery from even severe cases of Guillain–Barré syndrome, although some are left feeling weak. (The National Institute of Neurological Disorders and Stroke offers more information at: <www.ninds.nih.gov/disorders/gbs.htm>.)

A healthy immune system

When a doctor looks at the brain of a person with MS, the image or autopsy typically shows numerous scars in their CNS, especially in the white matter. Indeed, 'multiple sclerosis' means 'many scars'.[3] Essentially, these scars arise when your immune system mistakenly attacks myelin-encased nerves in the CNS.

Normally, your white blood cells help protect you from infections from bacteria, viruses, parasites and other pathogens. You produce several types of white blood cell, each with a different role, such as:

- producing antibodies (page 27);
- countering toxins produced by bacteria;
- engulfing and destroying the pathogen (harmful organism).

In addition, there are numerous subtypes of each of these white blood cells with specialist roles in our immune defences.

Signals released by cells switch the various white blood cells on and off. This allows the white blood cells to respond to a particular infection and target the damage in specific parts of your body. If you cut your finger, signals released by the damaged tissue attract white blood cells to the sliced flesh. The white blood cells don't home in on your big toe instead.

Autoimmune attack

Your immune system is exquisitely sensitive, capable of detecting subtle differences between the cells that are part of your body and those that indicate an infection or a cancer. This allows the immune system to tackle the infection, while sparing your healthy tissue. Occasionally, however, this process goes wrong: the immune system mistakenly attacks healthy tissue – a so-called 'autoimmune attack'.

If an autoimmune attack targets joints, you may develop rheumatoid arthritis. If it attacks your skin, you may develop psoriasis. If it attacks cells in the pancreas that produce insulin, you may develop type 1 diabetes. MS follows an autoimmune attack against myelin.

What goes wrong in MS?

So what triggers this autoimmune attack on myelin? Biologists are still working out the details, but a broad outline is beginning to emerge.

In most parts of the body, your blood vessels contain gaps – a bit like regular alleys in rows of terraced houses – that allow nutrients, cells and waste substances to move from and into your blood. Your body needs to protect your brain from harm, however, so the walls of the blood vessels that supply the brain and spinal cord have many fewer gaps than those in the rest of the body. Think of a wall around a country house: there's only the occasional gate. This 'blood–brain barrier' keeps harmful substances, organisms (such as bacteria) and blood cells out. When damaged or infected, however, the brain releases signals that open the gaps in the blood–brain barrier and allow white blood cells to pass into the brain.[3]

The blood–brain barrier seems to become abnormally leaky early in the 'natural history' of MS, possibly triggered by subtle changes to the brain. Indeed, the blood–brain barrier may become damaged before any noticeable changes appear on brain scans or symptoms emerge.[6] Radiologists can image this 'leakiness', which helps diagnosis (page 38). In people with MS, the influx of white blood cells attacks and destroys myelin.

Attracting the immune system's attention

White blood cells sometimes enter the CNS to fight infections without causing long-term harm, so why does myelin attract the immune system's attention in people with MS?

The details and order of events still need to be fully worked out. Essentially, however, MS probably arises from a mistake. White blood cells 'look' for certain proteins (called antigens) on, for example, a bacterium, or infected or cancerous cell. The rest of the body does not express these antigens, so white blood cells can home in on and destroy the invader or abnormal cell.

Hijacking cells

For instance, as we will see in Chapter 2, researchers believe that certain viruses influence the risk of developing MS. Viruses reproduce by hijacking a cell. They take the cell over and turn it into a factory for making more viruses. To complete their life cycle, viruses often change the proteins on the surface of the infected cell.

These altered proteins may be essential for the virus, but they also allow the immune system to home in on the infected cell. However, viruses and the immune system engage in an arms race. The virus adapts by making the surface proteins more like those on a healthy cell. This means that the virus can hide from the immune system. In turn, the immune system responds by becoming more sensitive to differences, but if the proteins are too similar, the immune system can damage healthy tissue.

In people with MS, a virus may 'activate' white blood cells outside the CNS, so the white blood cells home in and destroy infected cells. As we've seen, the blood–brain barrier of people with MS is especially leaky and the activated white blood cells enter the CNS. Unfortunately, the myelin of people with MS seems to express proteins that are very similar to those on the cells infected by the virus. As a result, the immune system 'mistakes' the myelin for the infected cells, which generates considerable inflammation and destroys the nerve.[6]

Some environmental factors (see Chapter 2) and certain genes interact to produce the protein that triggers white blood cells to attack the myelin and produce the signals that open the blood–brain barrier. In addition, MS flares from time to time. Some people find that certain factors – such as stress and infections – can trigger inflammation in the brain and lead to a relapse. Everyone's triggers are different. You might try noting what happened in the days before a relapse to see if you can identify your triggers.

The immune system usually clears an infection, so the white blood cells are no longer activated. This limits the collateral damage to the healthy CNS. In contrast, the change to the myelin is permanent. As a result, the immune reaction is persistently activated.[18] Essentially, the immune system seems to 'think' that the person with MS is still infected.

The hallmark of MS

Loss of the myelin sheath – demyelination – that surrounds healthy nerves is the hallmark of MS. However, the autoimmune attack can directly inflame, damage and destroy the nerves themselves. Indeed, the loss of myelin seems to leave the nerves themselves more susceptible to autoimmune damage.[6]

The inflammation arising from the autoimmune attack eventually burns out, leaving scars formed largely from astrocytes. These scars block the signal from travelling along the nerves.[3] When the body cannot compensate for the blocked signal, the person may develop symptoms of MS. In addition, certain chemicals released by white blood cells can interrupt the flow of nerve signals – called conduction block – without necessarily destroying any more myelin. Conduction block is reversible, which seems to be one reason the symptoms and signs often improve (go into remission) after the inflammation has subsided.[6]

When an infection directly attacks myelin, the brain usually makes good the damage. In contrast, the autoimmune attack in MS leaves the CNS scarred for life. These chronic plaques (damaged, 'scarred' areas in the CNS) show persistent myelin loss. In some cases, oligodendrocytes attempt to repair the damage in MS, by wrapping new layers of myelin around the nerve (remyelination).

Remyelination can sometimes be extensive. However, the new myelin sheath tends to be thinner, more susceptible to autoimmune attack and with less distance between the nodes, so the signal has to make more jumps. This slows the signal.[3, 6] Why the normal repair mechanisms do not work properly in people with MS is another facet of this enigmatic disease that we do not really understand.[3]

Inside your brain

The symptoms of MS depend on where the scars form in the CNS, so it's worth taking a quick and somewhat simplified look at the roles played by different parts of the brain (Figure 2). This will help you understand why the various signs and symptoms of MS can emerge.

- The **brainstem** ensures that our basic biological functions – such as breathing, heart rate and swallowing – continue without us thinking about them, even when we are asleep. The brainstem also helps with vision, hearing, balance, movement, the sleep–wake cycle, alertness and keeping our body temperature constant.
- The **cerebellum** (which literally means 'little brain') controls the timing and patterns of movement, helps you keep your balance and aids coordination. In particular, the cerebellum stores patterns of muscle movements. You call on the cerebellum when you take part in sport, for example, or play a musical instrument.
- The **cerebrum** receives information from the rest of the body, including our senses. The cerebrum analyses the information, compares our current situation with our knowledge (including our experience, our formal education and what we have learnt in other ways) and decides if we need to take action. If we need to respond, the cerebrum sends messages to our muscles.

So movement difficulties in MS could arise from scarring in the cerebellum or cerebrum or in the pathways that carry the signal down the spinal cord.

The cerebrum consists of two 'halves', called hemispheres. Each hemisphere controls movement and other functions on the opposite side of the body. In most people:

- the **right hemisphere** recognizes shapes, angles, proportions, patterns, faces and so on, controls emotions, creativity and imagination, and is responsible for your awareness of your body;

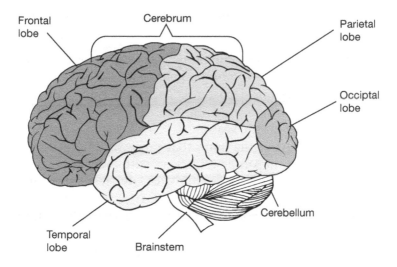

Figure 2 Some important areas of the brain

- the **left hemisphere** oversees analytical thought, problem-solving, language, speech and understanding.

A thick cord of nerves connects the two hemispheres. Each hemisphere has four lobes (Figure 2).

- The **occipital lobes** control and process vision.
- The **temporal lobes** form and store long-term memories and are important for hearing and understanding speech.
- The **parietal lobes** confer our sense of space and perspective, as well as receiving and interpreting information from our senses (such as touch and pressure) and contributing to speech.
- The **frontal lobes** influence personality, behaviour, decision-making, short-term memory and emotion, and are vital for movement and language.

Again, appreciating the different roles of the various lobes helps you appreciate why MS can be associated with such diverse symptoms (Chapter 3).

The many faces of MS

MS can affect different parts of the CNS, with different severity, at different times. The diversity of the autoimmune attack means that the signs and symptoms of MS can vary from person to person and within the same person over time.

- Damage to a part of the brain or the nerve pathways that control movement can cause 'motor problems', such as weakness, poor dexterity and abnormal postures. These can cause discomfort, which can range from mild stiffness to severe, uncontrollable and very painful muscle spasms.
- Damage to a part of the brain that processes information can cause 'cognitive impairment'. Those with MS and cognitive impairment are less able to think clearly, remember things, solve problems and plan, for example. They may lose keys and shopping lists, miss appointments or forget where they left their supermarket trolley or parked their car. We all do this from time to time, but this 'absent-mindedness' can become worse in a person with MS. Do not write the changes off – see your GP or tell your MS team. There are plenty of ways to give your mental abilities a boost (page 83).

Types of MS

Although MS varies widely, neurologists broadly divide the disease into three main subtypes:

- relapsing–remitting MS (RRMS)
- secondary progressive MS
- primary progressive MS.

There are several less common subtypes (page 18). For instance, a few people have a condition called 'benign MS'. Early on, benign MS seems identical clinically, on brain images and in blood tests, to the usual forms of the disease. Yet, over many years, people with benign MS do not develop any noticeable disability.[6] Why about 1 in 10 people with MS never develops progressive illness is yet another aspect that remains unclear.[6]

Relapsing–remitting MS

Almost 9 in 10 (about 85 per cent) of people with MS have RRMS.[3] From time to time people, with RRMS experience a worsening of their symptoms, called 'relapses', 'flares' or 'exacerbations'. We will look at these further on page 34. Relapses usually coincide with inflammatory changes ('lesions'), which are usually obvious to the MS team on MRI scans.

During a typical relapse, new or existing symptoms worsen for at least 24 hours and, more usually, a few days or a week. The worsening then plateaus for a few days. Finally, the symptoms steadily improve over a few weeks.[6] When there are no more symptoms, 'remission' has been reached. Treatment (page 42) can help relapses improve more rapidly, but does not seem to affect the long-term course of MS.

On average, a person with RRMS experiences one relapse every 2.5 years. However, the frequency of relapses varies widely between people with MS and changes over the course of the disease. Relapses tend to be common in early MS and usually become less frequent as the disease progresses.[6] Many treatments for RRMS seem to reduce the number of relapses (Chapter 5). This, in turn, delays the onset of disability. Unfortunately, the improvement between remissions tends to become less marked over time. Most people with RRMS eventually find that symptoms tend to persist between the relapses.[3, 6] In other words, they have developed 'secondary progressive MS'.

Short-lived exacerbations

People with MS may experience worsening of their symptoms, such as unpleasant sensations and muscle spasms, that lasts for a few minutes to several hours. These changes are too short-lived to be a full-blown relapse.

Rather than renewed autoimmune activity, these attacks seem to arise when a damaged area of the CNS becomes overstimulated. For example:

- some people with MS experience a sensation when they flex their neck that they compare to an electric shock – the movement seems to overstimulate the nerves;
- other people find that their symptoms worsen when their body temperature rises, leading to what doctors call Uhthoff's phenomenon,[6] which occurs because the increase in temperature 'short-circuits' the nerves,[19] and can make exercise difficult.

Secondary progressive MS

Sooner or later most people with RRMS develop secondary progressive MS. According to the MS Society, on average, about 13 in every 20 (65 per cent) people have developed secondary progressive MS 15 years after they were first diagnosed with RRMS.

In secondary progressive MS, people experience persistent symptoms and their disability gradually worsens. Typically, neurologists diagnose secondary progressive MS only if the disability clearly progresses over at least six months. A person with secondary progressive MS may still experience relapses, but will tend not to recover completely when the symptoms abate. In addition, recovery from the relapses can take longer than is usually the case with RRMS.

Eventually, secondary progressive MS can end in marked disability. As a very rough guide, those diagnosed with MS in their thirties will need a stick or cane, on average, 18 years later. They may need a wheelchair 25 years after diagnosis. The progression for a person with MS may be very different from these figures, however.[6] Some people only need a stick or wheelchair during a relapse and not while they are in remission.

Primary progressive MS

People with primary progressive MS experience a gradual building up of disability with no or minor relapses. The progression is apparent when MS is first diagnosed: they do not first experience a relapsing–remitting phase. Between 1 in 7 and 1 in 10 people with MS has primary progressive MS.[18]

According to the National Institute for Health and Care Excellence (NICE), neurologists should diagnose primary progressive MS only in people who show a progressive worsening over at least a year. Primary progressive MS tends to emerge at an older age than RRMS. Men are especially likely to develop primary progressive MS.[18] People with primary progressive MS generally decline more rapidly than those with RRMS.[6] The severity of the symptoms often fluctuates from day to day, but there is an inexorable decline, usually over several years.

Optic neuritis

About half of people with MS experience inflammation of the optic nerve, which carries signals from the light-sensitive retina at the back of the eye to the brain. Doctors call this inflammation optic neuritis.

Optic neuritis typically produces loss of vision in one eye and pain that gets worse when the person moves his or her eyes.[3, 6] Indeed, sight can be limited to a narrow band,[13] almost as if you were wearing a helmet. Other symptoms include:

- blurred vision
- blind spots
- double vision
- poor colour vision
- lack of contrast between light and dark.

In around 1 in 5 people with MS, symptoms arising from inflammation of the optic nerve are the first sign that he or she has developed MS.[3, 6] In addition, MS may change the way the eyes move. This seems to follow damage to the part of the brain that controls the eyes' movement.[13] MS occasionally leads to permanent loss of sight.

Clinically isolated syndrome

Your MS team knows only too well that being diagnosed with MS can be emotionally difficult and may affect your ability to drive, employment (page 90) and relationships. For these reasons, neurologists do not give a diagnosis of MS unless they are certain.

Several diseases can cause symptoms similar to MS (page 31). Because of this, doctors do not diagnose MS based on a single 'attack' of symptoms, known as 'clinically isolated syndrome'.[18] Although they may suspect MS, they tend not the make a formal diagnosis until you experience a relapse that is separated from the clinically isolated syndrome by at least 30 days.[6]

Although not knowing can be stressful, it is worth remembering that experiencing clinically isolated syndrome does not inevitably mean that you will develop MS. About a third of people with clinically isolated syndrome do not develop MS over the next 20 years.[6] The doctor should agree a date to review you and provide details of who to contact if new symptoms emerge or your current problems get worse.

Less common types of MS

Below are listed some less common types of MS.

- **Tumefactive MS** is characterized by a single large (more than 2-cm) ring-like area of scarring on the MRI. The lesion exerts pressure on the surrounding brain matter, which swells. Symptoms depend on the size and location of the lesion, but can include the following: speech and language difficulties; loss of the ability to recognize objects, faces, voices or places; seizures; and visual field defects. The symptoms typical of tumefactive MS are not usually seen in clinically isolated syndrome or RRMS.[18]

- **Marburg variant** (don't confuse this with Marburg disease, which is a viral disease similar to Ebola) is a particularly aggressive form of MS. Marburg variant can be fatal, sometimes even after a clinically isolated syndrome or the first relapse.[6]

- **Schilder's diffuse sclerosis** usually progresses gradually, although individuals typically experience periods during which their symptoms worsen. Schilder's diffuse sclerosis typically begins in childhood.[6]

- **Balo's concentric sclerosis** refers to an MRI scan that shows alternating concentric demyelinated and myelinated rings. Doctors have not linked this type of MS to a particular pattern of signs and symptoms.[6]

We will not consider these rarer forms of MS any further, but they underscore just how diverse MS really is.

2

The enigmatic causes of MS

As we've seen, MS arises when the immune system mistakenly attacks nerves in the CNS that are surrounded by myelin. Researchers are beginning to understand the fine details of this 'autoimmune attack', such as the particular types of white blood cells involved. Such insights help develop new treatments. What leads the immune system to attack the nerves remains more of a mystery. It is clear, however, that both genetic and environmental factors are at least partly responsible.

Nevertheless, tracing the environmental culprit is difficult. Over the years, doctors and CAM practitioners have linked numerous factors to MS, including:

- allergies and eczema
- certain chemicals
- glutens and dairy products
- insufficient blood flow to the brain – called chronic cerebrospinal venous insufficiency (page 53)
- mercury-containing dental amalgam used for fillings
- trauma or head injury
- vaccinations.

However, it's often difficult to disentangle cause from coincidence. Think of a businessman who wakes up sweaty, with a headache and a dry mouth after falling asleep in bed wearing his shoes. Wearing shoes in bed probably did not cause the perspiration, headache and dry mouth. It was probably the excessive drinking in the hotel bar the night before. This example seems obvious. However, distinguishing cause and effect from correlations (coincidence) is notoriously difficult, and researchers often use sophisticated statistical methods in very large numbers of people. In particular, numerous other factors may complicate the analysis. Our businessman may have passed out after contracting an infection or food poisoning, for example. He may have forgotten to turn the air conditioning off, then tripped, banged his head and knocked himself out. It's even harder if you need to assess the effect of a risk factor that happened many years ago or something common in the environment that only triggers the disease if the person also has certain genes. So it is easy to see why finding the environmental triggers for MS can prove difficult.

People with MS and vaccinations

Vaccination is one of the most important ways to protect your health and that of your family. Most studies suggest that vaccination does not increase the short-term risk of a relapse or the likelihood of developing MS.[6, 20] But if you experience a relapse that stops you from doing your normal activities or are otherwise unwell, it is probably better to delay vaccination. You may find it difficult to tell the difference between the relapse or another illness and a reaction to the vaccine. Indeed, it's easy to mistake urinary tract, respiratory (lung, throat and nose) and some other infections for a relapse.

Some MS treatments – including steroids used to treat relapses (page 42) – suppress the immune system. As a result, your doctor may advise against live (also called attenuated) vaccines if you are taking one of these drugs. Live vaccines contain weakened, but still viable, pathogens (such as a virus or bacterium). So you may be more likely to develop the disease the vaccine is supposed to protect you from. The shingles (herpes zoster) vaccine, for example, is a live jab. In contrast, the flu jab for adults is a killed (inactivated) vaccine. Although inactivated, the vaccine still contains the proteins that stimulate the immune response. In addition, make sure that the GP or nurse administering the vaccine knows which medications you are taking: for instance, some drugs that suppress the immune system may influence your response to vaccination. It's worth discussing vaccination with your MS team and reading the information on the patient groups' websites.

Cause or coincidence

The more people you examine, the more likely it is that a 'real' effect will emerge. A small study is more likely to show a spurious link simply by chance. One approach to distinguishing cause from coincidence – so-called meta-analysis – combines the results from several studies. For example, some people report trauma – such as a head injury – before the onset of MS or a relapse.[6] However, when researchers combined the results from several studies investigating the link, they found little clear evidence that trauma or injury increases MS risk.[20]

Unfortunately, many purported factors have been assessed only in small studies that differed in their design. So often there are not a lot of data to combine. We know that genes make an important contribution to the risk of developing MS. However, few studies take genetic make-up into account, although this is beginning to change. Such limitations make it difficult to totally rule out many

Is mercury linked to MS?

The CNS is especially sensitive to mercury poisoning. The tragic outbreaks of mercury poisoning in Japan during the 1950s and 1960s, the best known of which were in Minamata and Niigata, starkly illustrate the risks.

In 1956, for example, doctors in Japan recognized the first case of a cluster of symptoms that was eventually named 'Minamata disease'. Mercury released in waste from a factory contaminated the sea water. Most people who lived near to the factory ate large amounts of seafood and fish, which had absorbed the mercury. Many people who ate the contaminated seafood developed devastating symptoms, including paraesthesias (abnormal, unpleasant sensations such as tingling or pricking), changes in vision, movement problems, and difficulties hearing and speaking. Eventually, almost 3,000 people had confirmed Minamata disease. Nearly 600 people died during this outbreak of mercury poisoning in Minamata alone.[3, 22]

Many symptoms of mercury poisoning are similar to those of MS. However, MS is relatively uncommon in Japan, partly, ironically, because their diet is rich in fish and seafood. So any increase in the number of MS cases should be relatively obvious. Despite this, the Minamata tragedy did not seem to result in an increase in the number of people diagnosed with MS.[3, 22] Furthermore, when researchers combined several studies, they found little evidence of a link between dental amalgam and MS.[20] That said, mercury is incredibly toxic and there are alternatives. So while there is no firm evidence of harm, I've always avoided mercury-containing amalgam in fillings for myself and my family.

poorly studied but possible causes. However, most neurologists think that these probably do not make a major, if any, contribution to MS.[3, 20, 21] Instead, neurologists focus on genes, certain infections and vitamin D.

If you are worried about a particular risk factor, speak to your MS team or a patient support group. That's especially important if you are considering a complementary or unconventional treatment based on one of these correlations.

Genes

Your body contains trillions of cells. And almost every one of those cells contains an 'instruction manual' to make your entire body, contained in DNA's famous double helix. The amount of DNA in our bodies never ceases to amaze me. Pulled into a single, microscopically thin strand, the DNA would go from the Earth to the Sun and back more than 300 times, or wrap around the Earth's equator 2.5 million times.[23]

DNA is tightly packed into 23 chromosomes that contain the 25,000 or so genes that tell cells what to do and when. Genes determine your natural hair and skin colour, influence your height and weight, and build pathways that keep cells alive and working normally. Some genes influence your risk of developing certain diseases, including MS.

Studying twins

The strongest evidence linking genes to the risk of developing MS comes from studies that examined identical twins. As you may know, identical twins come from the same egg, which splits into two embryos in the first few days of pregnancy. So identical twins have identical genes (which is why it's so hard to tell them apart). Non-identical twins share half their genes, which is the same as siblings conceived at different times.

If MS were solely genetically determined, both identical twins would have the disease. If MS were solely an environmental disease, an identical twin would be no more likely to have the disease than a non-identical twin in the same circumstances. Most diseases – including MS – lie between these extremes: both environmental and genetic factors contribute. The genes make it more or less likely that you will develop a disease when exposed to the environmental factors.

Against this background, several twin studies underscore the contribution made by genes to MS.

- In a Canadian study, identical twins were about 200 times more likely to develop MS than the general population. By way of comparison, 1 in 3 (35 per cent) of the identical twins born to a person with MS and 1 in 29 (3.5 per cent) non-identical twins of a person with MS developed the condition.[3] The increased risk among non-identical twins compared with the general population reflects the fact that families share the same environment and many of the same genes, even if they are not identical twins.
- In an Italian study, about 1 in 7 (15 per cent) identical twins of people with MS also developed the condition.

Finding the genes responsible

By 2015, researchers had linked some 110 variations in our genes (the technical term is polymorphisms) to the risk of developing MS. Some polymorphisms increase the risk. Others reduce the risk. Together these variations seem to account for about a third (30 per cent) of the risk of developing MS.[6]

For example, biologists have linked an area on chromosome 6 known as the human leukocyte antigen (HLA) region with an increased risk of developing MS.[6] Most individual genetic variations have a relatively small effect on MS risk, but one variation – called HLA DRB1*1501 – roughly triples the risk.[24] (Don't worry about the name too much – biologists use it as a way to tell closely related genes apart.) Even so, most people who carry DRB1*1501 never develop MS and nearly half (45 per cent) of people with MS do not carry DRB1*1501.[6] This shows that environmental factors are also important. Interestingly, vitamin D seems to regulate the activity of DRB1*1501.[6]

Other genes also seem to contribute to MS. The vitamin D pathway involves numerous enzymes – proteins that speed up the chemical reactions that are essential for life. In the kidney, for example, an enzyme called CYP27B1 helps generate the biologically active form of vitamin D. A mutation in the gene that produces CYP27B1 probably accounts for about 1 in 500 cases of MS.[3]

- In the UK, about 1 in 4 (25 per cent) of the identical twins of a person with MS develops the condition compared with 1 in 23 (4.4 per cent) sisters and 1 in 31 brothers (3.2 per cent).[3]

In addition, certain genes seem to protect against MS or change the way in which the disease develops. For example, the Sami people – who live mainly by reindeer-herding – in Northern Scandinavia seem to carry genes that protect against MS.[3] MS is less common in people of darker skin than white people (page 3). When MS does arise, however, African-American people seem to develop a more severe form.[24] When MS develops in people of Asian origin, the disease predominately affects the optic nerve and spinal cord.[6] These different patterns seem to be, at least in part, genetically determined.[24]

Against this background, there is a small risk that you will pass genes that predispose to MS on to your children, but you should keep the risks in perspective. The risk that the son of a person with MS will also develop the disease is 1 in 167 (0.6 per cent), with 1 in 31 for a daughter (3.2 per cent).[3] If you are worried, speak to your MS team. A genetic counsellor can explain the risks.

Vitamin D

In 1922, the American biochemist Elmer McCollum identified a substance that prevented children from developing rickets – a disease caused by soft bones that was one of the scourges of Victorian society. Dickens may have had rickets in mind when he created Tiny Tim in *A Christmas Carol*.[25] At the time, the substance was the fourth known vitamin. So McCollum named the substance vitamin D.[4] Low levels of vitamin D contribute to rickets and osteomalacia (softening of the bones), falls and poor muscle strength and performance,[26, 27] difficulties that are also common in people with MS.

In addition, a growing number of studies suggest that vitamin D has numerous other health benefits (on reproductive health, heart disease, type 1 diabetes, cancers, asthma and, if you are pregnant, your developing child's brain development, for example).[26–28] Further evidence is needed to confirm many of these benefits, but people with MS can develop co-morbidities that include heart disease (page 2). In other words, the link between vitamin D and

MS goes beyond the risk of developing the disease itself. We will examine ways to get enough vitamin D to stay healthy on page 105.

The link with MS

There seems little doubt that vitamin D influences the likelihood of developing MS and possibly the risk of experiencing a relapse. For example:

- vitamin D reduces the number of some types of white blood cells that seem to contribute to the inflammation that causes MS;[4]
- low levels of vitamin D during critical growth periods could create weak and easily damaged myelin;[4] this may predispose children to damage if they experience an autoimmune attack;
- maternal vitamin D deficiency during early pregnancy seemed, in one study, to almost double (90 per cent increase) the risk of MS in their offspring compared with children of women who did not have low levels of vitamin D;[29]
- levels of vitamin D in the blood seem to be particularly low just before a relapse.[6]

Vitamin D deficiency is common

Unfortunately, many people – not just those with MS – show levels of vitamin D that are too low to protect the skeleton. (As many of the other actions are plausible but unproven, the official recommendations focus on skeletal health.) People at particularly high risk of vitamin D deficiency include those:

- with dark skin;
- from Afro-Caribbean and South Asian backgrounds;
- who are confined indoors (such as residents of care homes or some of those with limited mobility);
- who habitually cover their skin while outdoors.

In people with a white complexion, half an hour of sunlight produces 50,000 IU (1250 micrograms) of vitamin D.[30] So you'll get all you need before you burn, unless the sun is very strong. Nevertheless, according to the Scientific Advisory Committee on Nutrition (<www.gov.uk/government/publications/sacn-vitamin-d-and-health-report>), 3 or 4 in every 10 (about 30 to 40 per cent) people in the population have levels of vitamin D in their blood that increase their risk of bone disease in winter. The proportion falls in the summer, but between 1 in 50 and 1 in 8 (2 to 13 per cent) of us are still deficient in vitamin D during the summer.

Go north . . .

Vitamin D levels seem to explain why MS becomes more common the further you live from the equator. There are some important exceptions, which we will consider on page 103, but, in general, as sunlight gets weaker, you produce less vitamin D and the number of cases of MS rises.[31, 32] For example:

- even though the UK is relatively compact, MS is more common in Scotland than England;[4, 5]
- in the USA, for example, people living in Florida are about half as likely to develop MS as those in North Dakota, a mid-west state near the Canadian border;[6]
- people living on sunny mountaintops in Switzerland are less likely to develop MS than those in the valleys;[3]
- the protective effects of vitamin D seem to be especially marked on the rapidly developing CNS of children and teenagers (for instance, children who play outside are less likely to develop MS than those who remain indoors).[3]

Furthermore, in the northern hemisphere, people are slightly more likely to develop MS if they were born in May or June than the rest of the year. The risk is slightly lower if they were born in or around November. In the southern hemisphere, the pattern is reversed.

A mother pregnant during the summer gets plenty of sunlight and, in turn, vitamin D. And this seems to influence MS risk in children born a few months later. Incidentally, eating fatty fish (page 104) during pregnancy also seems to reduce the risk that the child will develop MS. (Fatty fish is a rich source of vitamin D,[3] although you may need to limit consumption of some fish during pregnancy – see page 103.)

Viruses

We tend to think of viruses as pathogens that cause deadly, debilitating infections, such as flu, AIDS, polio, hepatitis C or the current *bête noire* Zika, which can cause Guillain–Barré syndrome (page 8).

Viruses are everywhere, however: each millilitre of seawater, for example, contains about 10 million viruses.[33] Only a handful of the thousands of viruses known to science cause human diseases. Nevertheless, certain viruses contribute to the likelihood of developing MS or potentially trigger relapses.[6] For example, almost everyone reading this (90 to 99 per cent) has been infected with the Epstein–Barr virus (EBV), which seems to be associated with an increased risk of developing MS.[3, 6]

What is EBV?

EBV belongs to the herpes family of viruses. This family also includes sexually transmitted herpes and the pathogen that causes chickenpox and shingles. We usually catch EBV during childhood. EBV is transmitted in saliva, so previously uninfected teenagers commonly catch it by kissing.

In adolescents and older people, EBV can cause glandular fever (also called infectious mononucleosis), which is characterized by a high temperature, fatigue, a sore throat and swollen 'glands' in the neck. These unpleasant symptoms usually last 2 to 3 weeks, but EBV remains in our body for life.

Introducing antibodies

Antibodies, which are produced by some types of white blood cells, identify and help remove invading viruses, bacteria and other pathogens. Antibodies 'stick' to the microbe or infected cell, which allows the immune system to home in on the disease. Antibodies persist in the body so we mount a much more rapid immune reaction next time we encounter the same invader. (That's why vaccines protect against serious diseases.) So the pattern of antibodies in your blood can tell doctors what viruses, bacteria and so on you have encountered in the past. In addition, a growing number of drugs – including some for MS – are artificially created antibodies. These allow the MS team to hit a very specific target, such as a protein on the surface of a cell (page 146). These antibody-based drugs seem to reduce the risk of relapses, probably by interrupting the pathways that lead to inflammation and scarring.

EBV and MS

When researchers combined results from several studies, they found that people with antibodies to EBV were about 4.5 times more likely to develop MS than those without signs of the infection. Those who had suffered from infectious mononucleosis were about twice (a 117 per cent increase) as likely to develop MS as those who had not contracted this disease.[6, 20]

Differences in patterns of EBV infection may contribute to the variations in the number of people who develop MS worldwide. For example, almost every child in China has caught EBV by the age of six years. In contrast, at least half of six-year-old children in Scandinavia still have not been infected. MS risk is highest in parts of the world where people typically contract EBV later in life.[3]

Researchers estimate that being infected with EBV during adolescence or later life increases the risk of developing MS about 30 times compared with contracting the infection as a young child.[18] Nevertheless, the exact mechanism through which EBV contributes to the autoimmune attack underlying MS is not well understood.[6] Moreover, it is important to remember that not everyone who contracts EBV develops MS.

Smoking

Smoking increases the risk of developing MS by between a fifth and half (20 to 50 per cent)[6, 20, 34] and may mean that the symptoms progress more rapidly. In one study, for example, people who continued to smoke converted to secondary progressive MS at an average age of 48 years compared with 56 years among those who quit.[34] Smoking may influence the immune system, damage myelin and disrupt the blood–brain barrier, although, once again, the exact mechanism remains unclear.[20]

Helping you quit

In addition to slowing the progression of MS, quitting reduces your likelihood of developing most other smoking-related ailments, such as lung disease, certain cancers and heart disease. People around you who inhale your second-hand smoke are also more likely to develop several serious diseases, including cancer, heart disease, asthma and sudden infant death syndrome. So it is worth quitting if you already have MS, for the sake of both yourself and that of your family.

On some measures, nicotine is more addictive than heroin or cocaine. In part, nicotine is so addictive because of the withdrawal symptoms that emerge when blood levels fall, which include feeling irritable, restless and anxious, insomnia and intense cravings for a cigarette. Withdrawal symptoms typically abate over two weeks or so.

Nicotine replacement therapy

If you cannot tough it out, nicotine replacement therapy (NRT) 'tops up' levels and reduces withdrawal symptoms, without exposing you to other harmful chemicals. NRT increases your chance of quitting, but you need to find the combination that works for you. Patches alleviate withdrawal symptoms for 16 to 24 hours, but begin to work relatively slowly. Nicotine chewing gum, lozenges, inhalers and nasal spray act more quickly, but do not last as long. Talk to your pharmacist or GP to find out which is right for you. Doctors can prescribe other treatments, such as bupropion and varenicline, that help you quit.

Electronic cigarettes

Electronic cigarettes (vaping) can also help you quit. The nicotine staves off withdrawal symptoms and means you are not exposed to the chemicals that cause cancer and other diseases linked to tobacco. The wide range of e-cigarettes means that you should be able to find one that suits you. However, e-cigarettes can cause mouth and throat irritation and any long-term side effects are poorly characterized, so it is best to use e-cigarettes to stop rather than replace smoking.

Stay motivated

NRT and e-cigarettes help you quit, but you also need to be motivated and tackle any issues that maintain your habit. For example, smoking seems to offer some smokers a 'sense of control' and a way to 'fill a void created by a lack of meaningful activities'.[35] So keep a diary of situations that tempt you to light up – such as stress, boredom, a low mood, anxiety and worries, coffee, meals and pubs. Then find an alternative. If you find yourself smoking when you get home in the evening, for example, try a new hobby. If it is pressure at work, anxiety or depression, try mindfulness (page 93), meditation (page 93) or progressive muscular relaxation (PMR; page 95). If you find car journeys boring without a cigarette, try an audio book.

Here are a few other hints that may make life easier.

- Hypnosis (page 121) can increase the chances of quitting smoking almost fivefold.[36]
- Not letting other people smoke in your home helps strengthen your resolve.
- Try to quit abruptly. People who cut back the number of cigarettes usually inhale more deeply to get the same amount of nicotine. Reducing the amount that you smoke takes you a step towards kicking the habit.
- Set a quit date. Smokers are more likely to quit if they set a specific date rather than saying, for example, that they will give up in the next two months.
- Smoking is expensive. Keep a note of how much you save and spend at least some of it on something for yourself.
- Get a free 'Quit Kit' and other support online (at <www.nhs.uk/smokefree>) or call the NHS Smokefree National Helpline (0300 123 1044) to speak to a trained adviser.
- Your local stop smoking service offers support and advice, too. People who use the service with NRT are up to four times more likely to quit than those who just try to stop. Speaking to an adviser before your quit date can help you cope with withdrawal symptoms. Find your local service at <www.nhs.uk/smokefree/help-and-advice/local-support-services-helplines>.
- Watch your drinking. Abstinence from drinking seems to improve your chances of quitting. Alcohol can, after all, sap willpower.

3

Diagnosing MS

When she was 16 years old, the fourteenth-century Dutch Saint Lidwina of Schiedam (1380–1433) fell while she was skating. The fall was the first sign that she had weak legs. For the rest of her life, she experienced poor balance, weakness, headaches and changes in her eyesight. With the benefit of hindsight, neurologists believe Saint Lidwina had MS.[37]

As Saint Lidwina discovered, MS often emerges insidiously. You may notice a little dizziness, perhaps some pins and needles. You may feel more tired than usual.[1] A routine task may take longer – a symptom of the cognitive difficulties that MS can cause. Some people with early MS find, for example, that they need to take work home at the evenings and weekends. Despite this, they may make more mistakes.[2]

The MS mimics

Such experiences, of course, may have nothing to do with MS – which is why the disease can prove so difficult to diagnose. Depression, infections and stress, for example, can cause fatigue, weakness and poor concentration. If you're stressed and under pressure at work, you may find you need to work weekends and still make mistakes.

In addition, numerous other diseases can mimic the signs and symptoms of MS. That's one reason neurologists will not diagnose MS after a single attack of symptoms: the so-called clinically isolated syndrome (page 17).[18] Indeed, Scolding and Wilkins note that 'the range of disorders which *can* mimic multiple sclerosis is enormous' (italics in the original).[6]

The MS team will check for these other causes before stating that you have a relapse. Checking is more important today than it was in the past when there were fewer treatment options: today a relapse could trigger a change in your disease-modifying treatment or may be mistaken for a side effect of a drug. So your MS team will look for, in particular, infections and other illnesses that can mimic a relapse. They don't want to change a drug that is working.

A series of tests

As doctors cannot diagnose MS or a relapse accurately based on signs and symptoms alone, you will undergo a range of tests, which may include:

- brain scans
- blood tests
- lumbar puncture
- measuring the speed of nerve conduction.

The MS team may suggest other tests depending on your particular needs.

If you are diagnosed with MS, you will probably receive regular brain scans and other tests to track the progress of the disease, assess how well disease-modifying drugs are working and, possibly, monitor you for certain side effects. This information allows you and your MS team to consider when it is time to switch treatment.

Nevertheless, despite all the high-tech diagnostic tools, MS is notoriously variable. This means that the MS team cannot reliably predict your prospects. They will base their estimates on clinical studies that involve a large number of people and their considerable experience, but, obviously, the rapid advances in treatment mean that many of these studies are out of date. Some people with MS and their families find the uncertainty difficult to cope with,[3] which may be one reason for anxiety and depression being relatively common (Chapter 6).

In addition, you will have a lot of information to absorb when you receive a diagnosis. You will need to notify, for example, the DVLC, your insurance companies and, in some case, your employer. You should know these and other obligations as well as your legal rights, such as to social care, regarding employment and benefits. Your MS team, the hospital's medical social worker and patient groups can help.

Signs and symptoms

As we have seen, a network of nerves supplies every part of the body. So the signs and symptoms of MS depend on which nerves are damaged.[18] Table 1 summarizes some typical signs and symptoms. You will not necessarily experience every one of these symptoms.[3] And, of course, the number and severity can wax and wane as you experience relapses.

You should always let your MS team or GP know the full range and severity of your symptoms and any difficulties that you face in your daily life. Doctors base about four-fifths of their diagnoses on what patients reveal. However, when questioned after seeing their GP, 3 in 5 people had not disclosed some of their symptoms, because, for example, they felt that asking was inappropriate, or

Table 1 Examples of symptoms of MS

- Blurred or double vision; changes in colour perception; occasionally blindness
- Cognitive problems, affecting, for example, memory, learning and expressing yourself
- Difficulty swallowing
- Dizziness and vertigo, which can be accompanied by nausea and vomiting
- Fatigue
- Hearing problems, such as the words not seeming to make sense
- Loss of bladder control
- Mood and emotions, including developing depression and anxiety
- Muscle weakness and stiffness
- Numbness and tingling in the limbs (peripheral neuropathy)
- Persistent pain
- Problems maintaining balance
- Problems walking
- Sexual problems
- Spasticity
- Speech problems
- Tremors

they feared a negative reaction, or felt hurried. Your MS team or GP cannot diagnose and treat you appropriately without a full picture. You might want to keep a diary to give your MS team the information they need to help you (page 35).

When is a relapse not a relapse?

According to neurologists, a relapse of MS is characterized by one or both of the following:

- persistent worsening of one or more symptoms;
- one or more persistent new symptoms.

A relapse emerges rapidly – over hours or a few days – and then reaches a plateau. Some relapses have relatively little impact on your day-to-day activities: you may feel a little uncomfortable, but you can still manage. Some relapses mean that you have to take things easy for a while at home and ask your family for a bit more help around the house. Other relapses may be more severe and in certain cases you may need a stay in hospital. In general, you recover from a relapse within two or three months. However, in some cases, as the MS Trust notes, recovery may take up to a year.

A change in any MS or new symptom may be a sign of a relapse. According to the MS Trust, however, changes in or new issues with the following most commonly indicate a relapse:

- bladder control (incontinence or problems passing urine)
- dizziness, balance and coordination
- eyesight
- fatigue
- memory and concentration
- mobility and movement
- numbness, pins and needles or pain
- weakness in a leg or arm.

The change in symptoms needs to last at least 24 hours before the MS team will consider diagnosing a relapse. Indeed, many MS teams tend to prefer to diagnose relapses only after the symptoms have persisted for several days. As mentioned above (page 15), some people with MS experience worsening of their symptoms that lasts for a few minutes to several hours. These short-lived exacerbations are not relapses.

In addition, symptoms must occur at least 30 days from the start of the last relapse (to ensure that the worsening really is another relapse), and there must be no other explanation. For example, heat, stress, infections (especially urinary tract and respiratory infections) and several other factors can make symptoms worse and can be mistaken for a relapse. The team calls a worsening of symptoms that is not caused by MS a 'pseudorelapse'. Dealing with the underlying condition – such as using antibiotics to treat the infection – improves the symptoms of a pseudorelapse but will not help a true MS relapse.

A tough call

No two relapses are exactly alike, and deciding whether a new symptom or a worsening of an existing difficulty represents a relapse can prove difficult even for experienced neurologists and MS specialist nurses. (In many hospitals, MS specialist nurses rather than neurologists manage relapses, but the MS team members and their responsibilities depend on local arrangements and the severity of your symptoms.)

At your regular appointment, the MS team will probably ask – or you can volunteer – whether you have experienced new or worsening symptoms and when they occurred.[6] It is easy to forget, even if you don't have any cognitive difficulties. So:

- jot your symptoms down, keep a diary or use a smartphone, computer or tablet app;
- keep a record of any drugs you are taking (including painkillers and other drugs bought without a prescription), the doses and how often you take them;
- try ranking each symptom on a scale of 0 (not present) to 10 (the worst you have experienced or can imagine).

As mentioned below, however, it is important to contact your GP or MS team as soon as you suspect you might be experiencing a relapse.

Ask the family

Some symptoms – such as emotional or personality changes, and alterations in memory – may be more apparent to family and friends than the person with MS, so family members could raise any concerns with the MS team.

Equally, the full impact of MS may be apparent only to the person and the MS team. Pain is, for example, simultaneously, a universal human experience and deeply, intensely personal. Almost everyone agrees that hitting your thumb with a hammer hurts. However, the severity of pain each of us perceives and our responses vary, so it can be difficult to communicate the severity and impact of pain or 'pins and needles'. Likewise, the devastation that depression and anxiety can leave in their wake is impossible to appreciate unless you have also been unfortunate to experience the disease. Unfortunately, this might mean that some family members and colleagues feel that the person with MS is exaggerating or imagining the symptoms.[3]

When to seek help

The MS Trust suggests that if you are not sure if you are having a relapse, you could wait a day or two to see if your symptoms improve, but don't wait too long as, if you are, treatment needs to begin promptly (see page 43). Always contact your MS team or your GP if you think you are having a relapse, even if you do not think you need any additional treatment. Your MS team will look at your pattern of relapses to better understand the underlying activity of the MS, which may influence the choice of disease-modifying therapy. The MS team should provide details of who to contact if new symptoms emerge or current ones get worse. If you do not know, ask your MS team who to call.

Diagnostic issues

In general, a person will have developed damage in at least two places in their CNS before the neurologist will diagnose MS. For example:

- an MRI may reveal two distinct areas of damage;
- the person may experience two different symptoms;
- the person may experience two flares of the same symptom.

To diagnose MS, the symptoms or the lesion on MRI should occur repeatedly at least a month apart and the team needs to rule out other possible causes, such as infections.[3] You will therefore probably have a blood sample taken to test for other conditions and to evaluate how well your liver and kidneys, for example, are working. These tests can influence the choice of treatment.

Rating scales

The MS team may use 'rating scales' to ascertain the impact that MS has on your life and the severity of your symptoms. This helps them tailor management to you, determine the severity of the relapse and track how well treatment is working. The rating scales are also widely used in clinical trials of new treatments.

One of the most widely used rating scales, the EDSS (Expanded Disability Status Scale), measures the extent to which MS interferes with your life. The EDSS ranges from 0 (normal) and 1 (no disability) to 9 (confined to bed) and 10 (death).

The MS team may use other scales. The MSIS-29 (Multiple Sclerosis Impact Scale) uses 29 questions to look at, for example, arm and leg function, balance, coordination, bladder control, mental state, feelings and the impact that MS has on your social and leisure activities.[3] Other rating scales consider specific issues, such as depression and anxiety, bladder function and your general quality of life. In addition, the MS team may ask you to perform tasks that allow them to ascertain your ability. They might, for example, see how long it takes you to walk 25 feet (7 metres).

Neuroimaging

The introduction of MRI in 1981 revolutionized doctors' ability to diagnose and monitor MS and offered new insights into this enigmatic disease. For the first time, doctors could follow the activity of MS in a living brain. Before MRI, many insights into the causes and progression of this disease came from autopsy studies of the brains of people with MS who had died.

For example, MRI shows that MS can be active even when you do not experience symptoms.[37] The brain still shows areas of inflammation and nerve damage, but your body compensates. That's one reason why it is so important to take your medicine as suggested by your MS team and not just when you feel unwell. Regular treatment helps control the underlying autoimmune disease.

Plaque patterns

In people with MS, MRI reveals areas called plaques (also known as lesions), which are caused by demyelination, inflammation and loss of the nerve and other supporting cells.[18] Plaques can take several forms.

- Active lesions show myelin degradation and inflammation. Active lesions are particularly common in people with RRMS. The nerves themselves are usually relatively undamaged.[18]
- Chronic (also called inactive) plaques are more common in progressive MS than RRMS and generally show more extensive demyelination than active lesions. Chronic plaques also show marked damage to the nerves and oligodendrocytes (page 7), but in contrast to active lesions relatively little ongoing inflammation.[18]
- Some plaques show thinly remyelinated nerves and increased numbers of cells that develop into oligodendrocytes.[18] This seems to reflect the body's attempts to repair the damage caused by MS.

A radiologist (a specialist who takes images using X-rays, MRIs and so on) may inject a chemical called gadolinium into your bloodstream. As mentioned on page 10, the blood–brain barrier keeps chemicals and cells from entering the CNS. So, in a person without MS, an intact blood–brain barrier keeps gadolinium out of the CNS, but the blood–brain barrier tends to leak even in early MS. As a result, gadolinium will enter the brain, which shows up clearly on the MRI.[3]

Although MRI offers important insights into the disease, NICE says that neurologists should not diagnose MS based on brain scans alone. You may also have a brain scan if your MS team suspects that you might have, or are at high risk of, certain side effects, including progressive multifocal leukoencephalopathy (PML; page 40).

MRI and relapses

Studies using MRI suggest that damage to the brain from MS is about ten times more common than the relapses that cause signs and symptoms. In other words, not all the damage seen on an MRI scan causes a worsening of symptoms.[3]

A normal MRI does not rule out MS, however. Nevertheless, a lesion that shows demyelination is the most important predictor of a relapse in people with clinically isolated syndrome.[18] For example, 5 to 7 in every 10 people with a clinically isolated syndrome show several lesions in their white matter (page 7). More than four-fifths (82 per cent) of these develop MS in the next five years. By way of comparison, the risk in people with a normal brain scan is between 1 in 17 and 1 in 4 (between 6 per cent and 24 per cent) over the next five years.[6]

The changes in the brain scan are sometimes quite subtle and need an experienced neurologist or neuroradiologist (a radiologist who specializes in brain scans) to pick them up. In addition, conventional MRI is less able to examine grey matter lesions than those in the white matter. However, damage to grey matter may cause some features of MS, such as cognitive impairment.[6] So the MS team considers the brain scan alongside your signs and symptoms as well as the result of other tests.

Cerebrospinal fluid analyses

A clear, colourless liquid called cerebrospinal fluid (CSF) surrounds the brain and spinal cord. CSF cushions the brain and spinal cord from injury as well as providing nutrients and supporting a healthy CNS. Your neurologist may suggest a lumbar puncture (spinal tap) to take a sample of your CSF. A laboratory analyses the CSF for changes that indicate inflammation and damage to the CNS, such as the presence of 'oligoclonal' antibodies.[3]

Oligoclonal antibodies can appear in the CSF for several reasons other than MS. However, more than 19 in every 20 people with MS (95 per cent) produce oligoclonal antibodies in their CSF.[3] Oligoclonal antibodies do not seem to be present in the blood of people with MS.[6] In many other diseases that trigger a rise in oligoclonal antibodies (such as certain infections), however, they are present in both the CSF and the blood.

In some cases, a neurologist may suggest a lumbar puncture to measure levels of John Cunningham virus (JCV) in the CSF. As mentioned below, large amounts of this common virus are potentially associated with PML, a serious side effect of some disease-modifying treatments.

Progressive multifocal leukoencephalopathy (PML)

JCV was discovered in 1971. Between 7 and 9 in every 10 people worldwide have been infected with the virus. Most people catch JCV during childhood[38] and do not even notice, but it can lurk undetected in several parts of the body, including the kidneys, lungs, spleen, bone marrow, tonsils and some white blood cells.[39]

Sometimes this 'latent' JCV becomes 'active', moves into the brain, and selectively infects oligodendrocytes and astrocytes. This can trigger demyelination and, in turn, a potentially fatal condition called PML. In some people, PML causes symptoms that resemble MS or other neurological conditions.[39, 40] In other cases, PML is only apparent on MRI, which can create difficulties with diagnosis.

Several disease-modifying therapies used to treat MS seem to cause PML, which can also arise in people with HIV and those with certain blood cancers. Although it is relatively rare, the risk of PML rises with, for example, higher levels of JCV in the CSF and with the length of treatment with disease-modifying therapies. Even if you are high risk, however, you may not need to stop treatment. You can undergo regular brain scans that can detect the early signs of PML – which shows some subtle differences from a relapse. This allows the MS team to treat PML rapidly, should you develop it. So it is worth discussing the risks and benefits fully with your MS team.

Other tests

Your neurologist may suggest additional tests, such as evoked potential studies and other measurements of the speed of nerve conduction. These can help detect lesions in the visual pathways, brainstem or spinal cord that are not causing symptoms.[18] As we have seen, the myelin sheath ensures that nerves carry signals effectively. Normally, nerve signals travel along optic nerves at up to 400 km an hour (about 250 miles an hour), but the speed is lower in people with MS. By considering the results of these and other tests, neurologists and the team can diagnose MS, gain an insight into how severe it is and find the right treatment for you.

4

Drugs for MS

For decades, researchers have been searching for a treatment that will slow the progression of MS. By 1935, some 158 potential MS treatments had been tried. Nevertheless, in 1930 Russell Brain, a famous British neurologist, commented that 'the multiplication of remedies is eloquent of their inefficacy'.[37]

That changed in 1995, with the launch of interferon beta-1b. I covered the launch when I was working on a medical magazine and the excitement among both patients and neurologists was palpable. Unfortunately, much of the debate focused on the cost of treatment rather than its ability to transform the lives of people with MS. As I wrote at the time, the debate reminded me of Oscar Wilde's definition of a cynic as someone 'who knows the price of everything, and the value of nothing'.

Today, individuals with RRMS and the MS team can choose from several disease-modifying treatments that reduce the frequency of relapses. In many cases, disease-modifying treatments delay the emergence of disability. As disability usually takes several years to develop, some disease-modifying treatments have not been around long enough for us to see yet if they affect disability. In people with RRMS, however, disease-modifying treatments seem to reduce the risk that disability will progress by, on average, just over a quarter (28 per cent) compared with an inactive placebo (page 112).[41]

The wide choice of disease-modifying treatments means that MS teams and people with MS can think about what happens if the current treatment should fail. This is one reason why it is so important to let your MS team know when you experience a relapse: it might suggest that it is time to think about a different disease-modifying treatment.

Nevertheless, disease-modifying treatments do not work in everyone. If they do work, you will still probably experience relapses (although these will probably be less frequent than they would otherwise be). You may also experience side effects. All these things mean that it is important to understand the risks and benefits of each treatment. We will look at some questions you can ask your MS team later in the chapter.

A growing choice

In addition to those already on the market, numerous disease-modifying treatments are in development, especially for RRMS. And countless studies are underway with existing disease-modifying drugs that are helping the MS team tailor treatment better to each person. Indeed, as I was writing this chapter, another new treatment – an injectable drug called daclizumab – was approved to treat RRMS in adults. There are, however, far fewer options for people who experience progressive MS than are available for RRMS.

Each disease-modifying treatment has a distinctive pattern of benefits, limitations and side effects. You should speak to your MS team and check the websites of patient information groups to stay up to date. So, rather than explore the pros and cons of each drug, this chapter aims to offer a broad introduction to disease-modifying drugs and corticosteroids, which help speed recovery during a relapse. We will look at approaches that can help relieve specific issues, including fatigue, spasticity, bladder symptoms and pain in the next chapter.

Corticosteroids

In 1930, American researchers isolated a substance, which they called cortin, from the adrenal glands. (These glands lie on top of the kidneys and also produce, for example, adrenaline.) The researchers discovered that cortin contained a cocktail of hormones – now called the corticosteroids – that have several important biological actions, such as:

- controlling the way in which our bodies use carbohydrates, such as starch and sugar; carbohydrates are our main source of energy;
- regulating the balance of minerals and electrolytes (salts) in the blood;
- regulating the amount of fluid in the body;

- reducing inflammation, so drugs based on corticosteroids are used to treat numerous diseases, including asthma, eczema, arthritis and MS.

Doctors first started using steroids to treat MS relapses during the 1960s.[6] Initially, they prescribed a naturally occurring chemical called adrenocorticotropic hormone, which increases the production and release of cortisol, an anti-inflammatory hormone produced by the adrenal glands. You may know cortisol as hydrocortisone, its name when used as a medicine, such as in creams to treat eczema.

Man-made corticosteroids replaced adrenocorticotropic hormone in MS management during the 1980s. Today, your MS team may offer a course of steroids if a relapse produces marked difficulties, such as with your vision or movement. Steroids help your symptoms improve more rapidly by reducing the inflammation around the area of nerve damage. Unfortunately, steroids do not seem to change the level of recovery after the relapse resolves, or affect the long-term course of MS.

Taking steroids

When you experience a relapse, your MS team may suggest that you take a steroid tablet – usually methylprednisolone – for five days. They may suggest treating some relapses with injections or infusions of steroid directly into your blood if, for example:

- oral steroids did not work adequately during a previous relapse;
- oral steroids caused unacceptable side effects during a previous relapse;
- the current relapse is especially severe.

Treatment with intravenous steroids typically lasts between three and five days.

NICE suggests beginning treatment with steroids within 14 days of the start of the relapse – which is one reason why you should tell your GP or MS team as soon as you suspect you might be having a relapse. Some GPs and other healthcare professionals may not appreciate that you need a particularly high dose of steroids (typically 500 mg a day). The dose used to treat a relapse of MS is typically much higher than that used to help a serious exacerbation of, for example, asthma. Some MS teams provide a card that displays the recommended treatment, which you can show to other healthcare professionals.

A diverse group

Steroids are a very large group of natural and synthetic chemicals – which includes the corticosteroids used to treat MS and other inflammatory diseases as well as the sex hormones oestrogen, progestogen and testosterone. As this diversity suggests, steroids produce a wide range of effects on the body. For instance:

- one group of steroids, called mineralocorticoids, controls the body's use of minerals and electrolytes;
- another group, glucocorticoids, regulates levels of glucose in the blood;
- anabolic steroids are chemical relatives of testosterone, and are used medically to increase muscle mass and enhance physical performance.

Importantly, the corticosteroids used to reduce inflammation produce different effects from those produced by the anabolic steroids abused by some weight-lifters, athletes and body-builders. So you won't start putting on muscle or develop other side effects linked to anabolic steroids if you take corticosteroids for a relapse of MS.

Steroid side effects

Nevertheless, all drugs can cause side effects – even drugs in family medicine boxes can cause potentially fatal side effects. For example, paracetamol can damage the liver, and aspirin can cause bleeding in the gut. And steroids are no exception (Table 2).

NICE, for example, notes that the high doses of steroids used to manage MS relapses can cause temporary effects on mental health – such as depression, confusion and agitation – so you should watch for signs of these and other mental health changes and let your MS team or GP know, especially if they affect your daily life. High doses of steroids may also undermine the control of blood glucose in people with diabetes, so you might need to monitor your blood glucose levels more regularly. You should also let your MS team know if you are or could be pregnant before taking steroids to treat a relapse.

Table 2 Examples of side effects linked to steroids

- Acne (especially with long-term treatment) or rash
- Swollen ankles
- Cataracts (clouding of the lens in the eye) with long-term use
- Chest pain
- Diabetes with long-term use and poor blood glucose control
- Difficulty sleeping (insomnia)
- Flushing (especially in the face)
- Gastrointestinal symptoms, such as indigestion
- Headache
- Hypertension (dangerously high blood pressure)
- Increased appetite and, with long-term use, weight gain
- Metallic taste
- Mood changes (euphoria, restlessness, anxiety or depression)
- Osteoporosis with long-term use
- Palpitations (faster than normal heart rate)

Reducing steroid side effects

You may be able to reduce the chance that some of these side effects will develop. For example, taking the steroid with food may reduce the risk of developing indigestion. Taking the tablets in the morning may help if the steroid causes difficulties with sleep. Your MS team or GP may be able to suggest other solutions if you develop particular side effects.

To prevent long-term side effects (Table 2), many MS teams do not prescribe more than three courses of steroid a year to each person. (This isn't an issue for most people with MS. As mentioned above, however, on average, a person with RRMS experiences one relapse every 2.5 years.[6]) The MS team will prescribe steroids at the lowest effective dose for the shortest time possible.

If you have been on high-dose steroids for a while, doctors will gradually reduce your dose – so-called tapering. In general, however, the side effects produced by steroids are mild and resolve when you stop treatment.

Disease-modifying treatments

Since the introduction of interferon beta more than 20 years ago, several other disease-modifying treatments have become available for people with RRMS – and more are on the way. And there is no doubt that they can transform the lives of many people with RRMS. Indeed, many neurologists now believe that treatment with disease-modifying drugs should begin as soon as possible after the diagnosis of MS.

In RRMS, interferon beta and another disease-modifying treatment called glatiramer acetate, launched in the early 2000s, reduce the risk of relapse by just under a third (approximately 30 per cent). In other words, interferon beta and glatiramer acetate prevent, on average, one relapse every three years or so.[39] More recent drugs appear to be more effective. Natalizumab, for instance, reduces the risk of relapse by two-thirds (68 per cent), which is equivalent to preventing about one relapse every two years.[39]

Nevertheless, disease-modifying treatments do not completely prevent relapses or halt the progression of MS, and their effectiveness for you may be better or worse than these average figures suggest. It is important to have realistic expectations of disease-modifying treatment, so discuss the benefits and risks with your MS team. You will also need to take the disease-modifying treatment even when you feel better. As mentioned above, the autoimmune attack that causes MS can continue even when you do not experience symptoms.

A wide choice

All disease-modifying treatments for MS dampen the autoimmune reaction that attacks myelin. They differ, however, in the way they act. Some mechanisms of action are complicated and, in certain cases, are not fully understood. Even non-specialist healthcare professionals can have trouble understanding the details, so we will not consider the mechanisms of action here. If you want to know more, ask your MS team or check out the patient group websites.

In addition, disease-modifying treatments differ in terms of:

- how often you're treated;
- whether they are taken by mouth, self-injected at home or infused in hospital or sometimes at home;
- their side effects and other restrictions.

This may seem a lot to think about – but it means you have a degree of choice. Your neurologist or MS specialist nurse will discuss the options to find the right drug for you. As we will see later in the chapter, it is essential to follow your MS team's advice to gain the most benefit. Even the most effective drug will not work if you do not take it.

Differences in route of administration

You swallow some disease-modifying MS treatments – such as fingolimod, teriflunomide and dimethyl fumarate – as tablets or capsules. Other disease-modifying drugs are injected into a muscle (intramuscular injection; such as some forms of interferon beta) or under the skin (subcutaneous injection; other forms of interferon beta, for example). Others are infused into the bloodstream using a drip (for instance, natalizumab and alemtuzumab). (Natalizumab and alemtuzumab are both examples of antibodies used as a medicine.) Injections and infusions involve the use of a needle. Self-injection devices are easy to use and usually hide the needle, so most people soon become accustomed to self-injection.

Some people need an injection because this is the right choice for them at that time. Others prefer an injection once every week, fortnight or month to taking oral drugs more regularly. For example, dimethyl fumarate may need to be swallowed twice a day. Some people find that the regular treatment is an unwelcome reminder of their MS. In addition, some people who attend hospital for treatment find that talking to other people with MS offers a sense of community and they stay in touch outside the MS clinic. Have a full discussion to balance the various advantages and disadvantages of each method of administration.

In addition, several disease-modifying drugs are proteins. (That is why you can't take some by mouth – you would break them down in the same way you broke down your last meal.) The immune system sometimes recognizes these as foreign and creates antibodies against the disease-modifying treatment. These 'neutralizing antibodies' can stop the disease-modifying treatment from working. For example, about 1 in 17 people (6 per cent) develop neutralizing antibodies during the first six months of treatment with natalizumab.[42] A member of the MS team may take a blood sample to measure levels of neutralizing antibodies if, for example, you develop symptoms that might indicate a relapse.

Avoiding injection site reactions

Some people experience unpleasant reactions – such as pain, tenderness, warmth, itching, swelling and redness – around the site of injection. The tips given below may help.

- Do not inject in the same place; move the site around. As a rule, for example, you can inject subcutaneous disease-modifying drugs into fatty areas, such as thigh, buttocks, abdomen and upper arm. Ask your MS team or GP if you are not sure where you can inject.
- Wash your hands and clean the injection site to reduce the risk of infection.
- Some disease-modifying drugs need to be stored in the fridge. Allowing the medications to warm to room temperature before injection may be less uncomfortable than using colder drugs.
- Warm or cool the injection site for 30 to 60 seconds, which reduces swelling and pain.[43] Use ice or a warm pack.

What to ask your MS team

Before starting an MS treatment, fully discuss your treatment options with your neurologist or MS specialist nurse. Even if you do not want to question the team's suggestions, learning about the treatment and why it is right for you can help you understand the importance of sticking to their recommendations and how to prevent or deal with side effects. You should think about how the treatment will fit into your lifestyle. You may, for example, need to plan childcare and work around a treatment that is given in hospital.

Learn as much as you can about your treatment. You should know the medical name of any procedure (to help you look it up) or a drug's brand and scientific ('generic') names. For example:

- **alemtuzumab** is the generic name for the brand Lemtrada;
- **dimethyl fumarate** is the generic name for the brand Tecfidera;
- **fingolimod** is the generic name for the brand Gilenya;
- **natalizumab** is the generic name for the brand Tysabri.

Sometimes a medicine can have several brand names and different packaging. The generic name, however, remains the same; you need to look up both names. You should also read the patient information leaflet included in the package or online (<www.medicines.org.uk/emc/>) and speak to your doctor, nurse or pharmacist if you have concerns or questions.

Certain drugs interact with other medicines, foods, CAMs and drugs bought 'over the counter' from pharmacists and supermarkets. Read the patient information leaflet and tell your doctor and pharmacist if you are taking other medicines, conventional or complementary. For example, St John's wort (*Hypericum perforatum*) is best known as a herbal treatment for depression and anxiety. Combining St John's wort and selective serotonin reuptake inhibitors – a group of drugs prescribed by doctors for depression and anxiety – can trigger a potentially fatal condition called serotonin syndrome.[44] St John's wort can also interact with oral contraceptives, leading to unplanned pregnancies and breakthrough bleeding.[44] It is important, therefore, to tell your MS team and pharmacist about any treatment you are taking.

What to ask: a checklist

You and your family will inevitably have questions about MS and its treatment, but remembering everything you want to ask in the short time you have in the clinic can be difficult, so keep a notebook or use your smartphone to jot down any questions. Feel free to take notes and ask questions when you speak to the MS team. Taking a friend or relative with you helps you understand what you are discussing during the visit and can help refresh your memory afterwards.

The box (overleaf) includes some of the most important things to ask about any treatment – for MS or otherwise. You could photocopy, scan and print, or take a snap of the box on your mobile phone so that you can refer to it during the consultation.

If you don't take the drug, it won't work

As we've seen, the brain scans of people with MS can show damage even if they are not experiencing a relapse or their symptoms are getting worse. You take disease-modifying drugs not just to reduce

Questions to ask your doctor or nurse

☐ What is the goal of treatment (for example, trying to modify the course of MS or tackle a particular symptom?)
☐ Why is this the best treatment for me at this time?
☐ How does this compare with other treatments?
☐ What were the results of the main clinical studies? How similar were the patients in the study to me? (Sometimes a study may include a relatively restricted range of patients.)
☐ How and when will I know that treatment is working?
☐ How and when I know that treatment is not working?
☐ How will the treatment help me reach my goals?
☐ What are the risks, complications and side effects? How do these compare with other treatments?
☐ What symptoms should I watch for that might indicate side effects or complications?
☐ Will the treatment affect my quality of life for better or worse?
☐ What can I do to reduce the risk of side effects?
☐ Will I need to change my lifestyle or activities?
☐ What should I do if I miss a dose?
☐ What should I do if I accidentally take another dose too soon?
☐ Whom should I contact if I have any concerns or questions?

the frequency and severity of symptomatic relapses but also to reduce the number of lesions that do not cause symptoms as they can still drive the progression that can end in disability. That is why you should take the medicines as agreed with your MS team and never stop or reduce the dose without a discussion. Healthcare professionals call the extent to which you follow their advice 'adherence', 'compliance' or 'concordance'.

Good compliance seems to improve the prospects of people with MS. For example, a study of 1,606 people with RRMS found that, over a year, taking interferon beta as suggested by the MS team prevented about 1 in 10 relapses (11 per cent) and reduced admissions to hospital by a fifth (21 per cent).[45] In another study, people with RRMS who discontinued therapy showed greater disability and were more likely to experience relapses and progression than those who kept taking the disease-modifying treatment.[43]

Despite the undoubted benefits of treatment, poor adherence is relatively common among people with MS. In the study of 1,606 people with RRMS taking interferon beta, only between a quarter (27 per cent) and two-fifths (41 per cent) took at least 17 in every 20 (85 per cent) doses over a year. Just 1 in 25 (4 per cent) took at least 85 per cent of the doses over three years.[45] Likewise, only between three-fifths (60 per cent) and three-quarters (76 per cent) of people with MS adhere to interferon beta or glatiramer acetate for between two and five years. During a study that followed patients for eight years, half (49 per cent) of those who stopped disease-modifying treatment did so in the first two years.[43]

Why do people with MS not take their medicines?

People with MS may not follow their team's advice for several reasons.

- Some people find that self-injecting disease-modifying therapies is a burden. They may agree and adhere at first, but then become fed up with the treatment – so-called injection fatigue.
- For some people with 'needle phobia', injections may provoke fear, anxiety, palpitations, flushing and even disgust, so they may ask a family member to inject the drug. However, this can undermine the person's independence and may mean they miss injections when their carer is not available.[43]
- Many people do not experience a relapse or develop signs and symptoms for years or months after diagnosis, so they may not feel that they need treatment.[43] Ironically, the lack of signs and symptoms is often a sign that treatment is working.
- If symptoms do not abate with treatment, or new symptoms or relapses develop, some people feel that the treatment is not working so do not adhere to it. However, as mentioned above, it is important that you and your family have realistic expectations about treatment – even the most effective disease-modifying treatments do not cure MS.[43] Nevertheless, the growing number of disease-modifying drugs for MS means that a relapse is often a good time to discuss switching treatment.
- Some symptoms of MS make taking drugs difficult. If MS, arthritis or another problem affects fine movements, for example, you may find opening packaging and self-injection difficult. Your pharmacist and MS team can suggest several approaches that

might help you administer your treatment, such as repackaging the medicines in containers that are easier to open.

- Between 1 in 7 (14 per cent) and half (51 per cent) of people with MS stop treatment with some disease-modifying drugs because of side effects, such as flu-like symptoms, depression and injection site reactions.[43] You can often alleviate side effects. For example, painkillers may help flu-like reactions,[43] and the tips on page 48

Remembering to take your treatment

Remembering to take your treatment can be challenging, especially if you have several drugs to remember (including for ailments other than MS), you feel depressed and demotivated or you are experiencing cognitive issues. Try the following suggestions to help you with this.

- Ask your partner or carer to remind you to take your dose.
- Keep a checklist and cross off or tick each dose when you take it.
- Use an app that allows you to track your use of medicine.
- Leave yourself notes reminding you to take your treatment; you can put these on the fridge, over your desk, next to the TV, on the bathroom mirror, wherever works for you.
- If you do not have young children, grandchildren or pets (and the treatment does not need to be kept in the fridge), you could leave your medicines where they are easily seen, such as on the dining or bedside table or on your desk.
- Try to take your treatment at the same time each day, which helps build a routine. You could use an alarm on a watch, phone or timer to remind you.
- Your routine may change when you are on holiday, a day out, at a birthday or wedding, or away on business, so you may need to adjust your timings. Make sure you have sufficient supplies of all your medicines for the time that you are away.

Some people feel that alarms are intrusive and remind them they are ill. If the alarm goes off in public, you might not want to explain about your MS. You may feel irritated if carers remind you to take a medicine when you have already done so. If you share the app electronically or by pinning the list to the wall, your partner or carer only needs to remind you if you've forgotten. Try different things to find what works for you.

often reduce the frequency and severity of injection site reactions. You may be able to schedule the injections for days or times when the adverse events may pose less of an issue.[43] If you feel that you are developing side effects, speak to the MS team, who can often offer some suggestions to help.

- Depression, fatigue and cognitive symptoms – such as poor memory – can also undermine compliance.[43] Indeed, about half of the people with MS who do not follow their team's advice simply forget.[43] The box 'Remembering to take your treatment' (left) offers suggestions that might help.

Other treatments

In addition to drugs, some clinicians have tried a range of other treatments for MS, including stem cells, hyperbaric oxygen and treatments for chronic cerebrospinal venous insufficiency (CCSVI). For example, hyperbaric oxygen, which involves breathing through a mask in a pressurized chamber, is popular.[6] Some doctors have found that certain patients benefit from hyperbaric oxygen.[1] You could discuss this option with your MS team.

Stem cells can, in theory at least, diversify into numerous other cells, including those damaged in MS. Many biologists believe that stem cells could, in the future, prove a valuable treatment, and this is one of the most active areas of research in MS. Patient group websites can help you stay in touch with the exciting developments. The research is, however, at a very early stage, and the risk, the benefits and who might benefit isn't clear. If you want to try stem cell treatments, it is best to see if you can take part in a clinical trial. Speak to your MS team, who can find out if any trials of stem cells or other treatments are underway that might help you.

Cerebrospinal venous insufficiency

Some research seems to link MS with poor blood drainage from the brain and upper spinal cord – a condition called CCSVI. Some doctors therefore suggest treating MS by increasing the diameter of, and supporting, the veins using a metal mesh or a small balloon. (These approaches are more commonly used to treat the blocked blood vessels that can cause strokes and heart attacks.)

Social media posts often extol the benefits offered by CCSVI surgery. In one study, almost 9 in 10 (86 per cent) of people with MS on social media who had undergone the procedure reported that at least one symptom showed some improvement after the procedure. The most common message from people with MS is that treatment of CCSVI 'is not a miracle but worth trying'. Some healthcare professionals agree. Social media posts from healthcare professionals report that treating CCSVI may improve fatigue, cognition, pain and incontinence.[46]

Nevertheless, when researchers combined the results of investigations into CCSVI they found that the results were very variable and there was 'no clear scientific evidence to support the link' or that surgery helped.[20] CCSVI surgery has also been linked to potentially serious side effects (see <www.fda.gov/MedicalDevices/Safety/AlertsandNotices/ucm303318.htm>).

As with any treatment, it is essential you fully understand the potential risks and the weaknesses of the supporting data – as well as the purported benefits. You should also always bear the placebo effect – which can be considerable – in mind (page 112). If you want to have the operation privately – or indeed try any unproven treatment – fully discuss the risks and benefits with your MS team, the surgeon or doctor offering the procedure and a patient group.

5

Treating particular problems

People with MS often experience a wide range of symptoms and issues, and may, as a result, draw on the expertise of several healthcare professionals, including physiotherapists and physical therapists, occupational therapists, orthotics (external devices that support the body or prevent or assist movement), ophthalmologists, dietitians and neuropsychologists. This multidisciplinary team will devise a management programme that will help you remain as independent as possible for as long as possible.

The programme is tailored to your condition, your goals and your lifestyle, so the comments in this chapter are only guides. In addition, you should bring any difficulties or issues to the attention of your MS team. The challenges you face may vary over time, even if your MS symptoms are relatively stable. You may, for example, find that your lifestyle changes (such as having children or changing jobs) or you develop another condition. According to NICE, you should have a 'comprehensive review' that covers all aspects of your MS care at least once a year. However, as mentioned above, tell your GP or MS team if you develop new symptoms or existing ones get worse between routine appointments. These could indicate a relapse or a further progression.

As the programme is tailored to your particular case, the following are points that you could discuss with your MS team. Any advice they have overrides the suggestions in this chapter.

Pain

Between 40 and 80 per cent of people with MS experience chronic (long-lasting) pain (Table 3),[47] which seems to be especially common in progressive MS and can take various forms.[6] For example:[2, 48]

- many people with MS suffer paraesthesia; in other words, they experience unpleasant sensations, including tingling, tickling, pricking, burning and 'pins and needles';

- some people with MS report Lhermitte's sign, characterized by unpleasant sensations down the back and, sometimes, into the limbs when they bend their neck forward;
- others may experience trigeminal neuralgia, which is a sudden, severe, sharp and shooting facial pain.

Your MS team needs to understand the causes of your pain, such as those given below, to find the best way to help.

- Pain can arise from inflammation and scarring of the pathways that carry pain signals in the CNS. This can cause 'central neuropathic pain', which is typically described as a constant, burning-type pain in the lower limbs.
- Pain may arise from physical problems caused by MS, such as the stress placed on joints caused by walking difficulties.[6, 19] Some people with MS experience painful tonic spasms – cramping or pulling pains – especially in the legs. Spasms seem to be closely linked to spasticity (page 72).[6]

The pain can, of course, have nothing to do with MS. Always speak to your MS team if you experience pain or the discomfort is getting worse.

Table 3 Patterns of pain among people with MS[2, 48]

Form of MS	Proportion reporting pain
All people with MS	63% (3 in 5)
Primary progressive MS	70% (7 in 10)
Secondary progressive MS	70% (7 in 10)
RRMS	50% (1 in 2)
Type of pain experienced by person with MS	Proportion experiencing symptom
Paraesthesia	87% (9 in 10)
Headache	42% (2 in 5)
Pain in the extremities (e.g. hands and feet, e.g. peripheral neuropathy)	27% (3 in 10)
Back pain	20% (1 in 5)
Lhermitte's sign	17% (1 in 6)
Painful spasms	15% (1 in 7)
Trigeminal neuralgia	4% (1 in 25)

Keep a note

To help your MS team better understand your symptoms, you could keep a diary or use a smartphone to note the aspects given below.

• How bad was the pain? Try rating the pain on a scale of 1 (just apparent) to 10 (the worse you have experienced or can imagine).
• What did the pain feel like? Try to be specific. Was it dull and aching? Sharp and stabbing? Or did it feel like electric shocks or pins and needles?
• What was the impact on your life? Did the symptoms interfere with your plans, or stop you working or performing a normal activity?
• What you were doing when the symptom occurred? This helps you and the MS team identify and tackle factors that can trigger or exacerbate the pain.

Treating pain

Often simple painkillers (analgesics) – such as aspirin, paracetamol and ibuprofen – alleviate the pain. If these fail to adequately relieve your discomfort, your MS team may suggest a more powerful pain-killer. As painkillers can cause side effects, it is especially important to take these as suggested by the team. In addition:[2, 6]

• several drugs – some of which are used to treat depression and epilepsy – can alleviate neuropathic pain;
• surgery may help, for example, pain due to severe spasticity (muscle stiffness);
• several drugs – such as gabapentin, carbamazepine, baclofen and benzodiazepines – may alleviate painful spasms (page 72);
• pain associated with optic neuritis (page 17) is usually short-lived, but may benefit from steroids or non-steroidal anti-inflammatory drugs – the latter are drugs related to aspirin that reduce inflammation;
• many CAMs discussed in Chapter 8 – including acupuncture, hypnosis and yoga – can alleviate pain – some seem to directly reduce pain, such as by releasing the body's natural analgesics called endorphins, some help you relax: pain is always worse when you are stressed and some do both;
• regular exercise can help by keeping you mobile and releasing

endorphins and massage alone or combined with exercise seems to reduce pain more than exercise alone.

Fatigue

Up to four-fifths (80 per cent) of people with MS develop fatigue. Once again, fatigue is more common in progressive MS than RRMS,[6] although the pattern varies widely. Some people with MS find that the fatigue is worse at certain times of the day, whereas others find that the fatigue is relatively constant. Some find that the fatigue suddenly arises.[13] Nevertheless, two-thirds of people with MS regard fatigue as one of their most challenging symptoms.[2]

Fatigue in people with MS can have several causes.[3]

- People with MS often feel especially fatigued after exercise. After all, exercise can be especially hard for many people with MS.
- Depression and anxiety can create a sense of lassitude.
- Fatigue in MS might be a symptom of a relapse or an infection.
- Chronic pain, spasms, bladder symptoms and certain drugs can contribute to fatigue.
- Sleep disturbances can be caused by, for example, steroids (page 42). In particular, some steroid users experience difficulties falling asleep.

Identifying the factors that cause or exacerbate fatigue can help the MS team figure out the best way to help you. Often, however, the team cannot identify a particular cause for the profound, over-whelming fatigue experienced by certain people with MS. Some researchers believe that the CNS might be working especially hard to make up for the effects of the MS and the repair processes are in overdrive.[13]

This 'MS fatigue' can arise suddenly and without warning. The loss of energy can take you by surprise, leave you feeling dazed and unable to communicate. Your body, such as your arms and legs, may feel heavy. You may experience difficulties concentrating or thinking clearly. Indeed, severe fatigue may leave a person with MS unable to perform everyday activities that the rest of us take for granted, such as eating, shopping, working, exercising or even personal hygiene.[13]

Keep a fatigue diary

Other people often do not appreciate just how devastating MS fatigue can be, so keeping a diary helps you, your family and your MS team identify the causes and triggers. The diary also helps clarify the impact on your ability to perform the normal activities of daily living and on your quality of life. Understanding the triggers and consequences helps identify the best way to help you. Record the information given below in your diary.[49]

- When the fatigue arises. Many people with MS find that their fatigue follows a pattern, such as being most severe in the afternoon. This allows you to plan your time and pace yourself with rest periods.[19]
- The fatigue's severity. Try ranking severity on a scale of 0 for no fatigue or tiredness to 10 for the worst fatigue you've experienced or can imagine.
- How much the fatigue interferes with your daily life. You could rank this from 0 for no interference to 10 for being unable to get out of bed or out of a chair.
- Your sleep patterns and daily activities. This may help identify triggers and causes.
- What you did to try to address the fatigue and whether or not there was any improvement. You could rate the effectiveness on a scale of 0 for no improvement to 10 if the fatigue resolved.

Planning, prioritizing and pacing

The diary also helps with planning, prioritizing and pacing. Taking a proactive approach helps you to spend your time and energy on activities you value most. Try the suggestions given below.

- List things that you *have to do* and what you can leave or ask someone else to do.
- Make a list of who you can ask for help, for what and when (so that, for example, it fits in with their commitments). Family and friends are usually more than willing to help, but often do not know what to do or feel uncomfortable asking. They could help by, for example, giving you a lift to hospital, looking after the children, cooking or helping with the housework. Helping out will often make your family and friends feel better.

- Plan your daily routine, which should include regular rest and relaxation. You may find that you need to add extra rest before or after activity or visitors. Take a break if you feel you need to rest, even if it is unscheduled. Struggling on often just makes matters worse. Nevertheless, you need to strike the right balance between rest and activity. Excessive rest can sap your energy and interfere with sleep. Your diary can help you discover the balance that's right for you.
- Make time for exercise. Although it might not make immediate sense, exercise is a great way to counter fatigue.[2] NICE, for example, suggests that yoga (page 122) or other aerobic, balance and stretching exercises may help treat MS fatigue.

Your MS team can help you get extra support. For example, cognitive behavioural therapy (CBT) – one of the so-called talking therapies (page 91) – and mindfulness-based training (page 93), may help you cope with fatigue.[2] Some people benefit from help from an occupational therapist, who can help you plan your time, simplify your work and help you perform activities in the most effective manner.[19] NICE suggests that a drug called amantadine may alleviate fatigue in some people with MS.

Difficulties with sleep

Sleep is a basic biological need. Apart from leaving you grumpy and heavy-eyed, not getting enough sleep is linked to a range of health issues, including depression, being overweight and diabetes. For example, people with MS often experience disrupted night-time sleep and daytime sleepiness, which seem to increase pain, fatigue and depression.[50] Indeed, sleep disturbances seem to be more common in people with MS than the rest of the population and can arise from:[6]

- depression
- pain
- side effects, such as from steroids used to treat relapses
- spasticity
- urinary symptoms.

Pain and depression can contribute to sleep disturbances. They can also arise from sleep disturbances. It's easy to get caught in a spiral.

Tips for a good night's sleep

Speak to your MS team, as a change in your management some-times helps – such as taking steroids in the morning (page 45) if these could contribute to your sleep disturbance. In addition, you could try the following tips (many will also help if your partner also sleeps poorly).

- Although regular exercise during the day helps you sleep and counters fatigue, exercising just before bed can disrupt sleep.
- If you feel fatigued, schedule rest regularly throughout the day. However, try to avoid naps, which can make it difficult to sleep at night.
- Avoid alcohol. A nightcap can help you fall asleep, but, as levels of alcohol in your blood fall, sleep becomes more fragmented and lighter. This means you may wake repeatedly in the latter part of the night.
- Avoid stimulants, such as caffeine and nicotine, for several hours before bed. Try hot milk or milky drinks instead.
- Remain hydrated. Note, however, not to drink too much fluid (even non-alcoholic) just before bed as this can mean regular trips to the bathroom.
- Do not eat a heavy meal before bedtime.
- Keep a sleep diary for a couple of weeks to work out what time you need to go to bed and get up. Then go to bed at the same time each night and set your alarm for the same time each morning, even at the weekends. This helps re-establish a regular sleep pattern.
- Make the bed and bedroom as comfortable as possible. Invest in a comfortable mattress, with enough bedclothes, and make sure the room is not too hot, too cold or too bright.
- Do not worry about anything you have forgotten to do. Get up and jot it down (keep a notepad by the bed if you find you do this a lot). This should help you forget about the problem until the morning.
- Try not to take your troubles to bed with you. Brooding makes problems seem worse, exacerbates stress, keeps you awake and, because you are tired in the morning, means you are less able to deal with your difficulties. Try to avoid heavy conversations and arguments before bed. Indeed, try to make the last couple

of hours a time of calm: have a bath with some aromatherapy, for example.

- Use the bed for sex and sleep only. Do not work or watch TV.
- If you can't get to sleep, get up and do something – nothing too exciting or stimulating. Lying there worrying about sleeping can make matters worse.

Bladder symptoms

Bladder symptoms can be embarrassing, hinder your social life – you might worry about reaching the toilet in time – and keep you awake at night. However, about three-quarters of people with MS experience bladder symptoms, such as:[3]

- urinary incontinence: involuntary passing of urine;
- passing urine more often than usual;
- often feeling an urgent need to go to the toilet;
- excessive urination during the night (nocturia);
- feeling that your bladder has not emptied fully after urination;
- difficulties starting or maintaining urination (hesitancy).

These issues are often accompanied by bowel and sexual symptoms, and are particularly common in progressive MS.[6] Constipation also seems to increase the risk of bladder symptoms.[6]

Your MS team should ask about your bladder function, but always tell them if you develop any of these symptoms. Bladder issues

Watch for urinary tract infections

See your GP if you develop any of the following, which may indicate that you have picked up a urinary tract infection.

- You have urinary incontinence or retention (you cannot urinate).
- You urinate much more or less often than usual.
- Urination hurts or your lower back hurts.
- Your urine changes colour – such as being bloody or brown.
- Your urine smells.
- Your urine seems to have a different consistency from normal.
- Your urine seems to contain a sediment.
- You have other signs of an infection, such as chills or a fever.

often arise when inflammation and scarring of the spinal cord interrupts the signal between the areas of the brain that control urination and the bladder. As a result, bladder function may worsen during a relapse.

Bladder function can also worsen if you contract a urinary tract infection. Indeed, a urinary tract infection may mimic an MS relapse.[6] As steroids dampen the immune system, they can worsen urinary tract infections.[6] That's why the MS team should rule out a urinary tract infection before deciding that you have experienced a relapse.

Treating urinary symptoms

Ultrasound and cystoscopy help the team check for any underlying problem.[6] During cystoscopy, the healthcare professional passes a thin tube with a light and a camera at one end into the urethra, the tube that carries urine, and on into the bladder. The MS team can also measure (usually using ultrasound) the amount of volume remaining in the bladder after you urinate, which helps them determine how to help.

- If you have less than 100 ml of urine remaining after you 'empty' your bladder, you may have a condition called 'bladder overactivity'. Your MS team can prescribe drugs that might help, although, as always, these can cause side effects. Pelvic floor exercise and bladder training may also help an overactive bladder.[6] Your MS team can tell you how to do this or refer you to a nurse who specializes in bladder problems.

- If more than 100 ml of urine remains, you may not be emptying the bladder fully and you may need a physical method, such as a catheter, which you, a partner or another carer can learn to insert.[3,6] A catheter, however, may increase the risk of contracting a bladder infection. Some people with severe bladder symptoms may need a permanent catheter.

- Another approach injects botulinum toxin ('botox' – the same drug used to treat crow's feet and other 'wrinkles') into the bladder; this relaxes the muscles and, in turn, helps you pass urine.[3]

Bowel symptoms

Some people with MS experience changes in their bowel habits, usually constipation. These changes can reflect several underlying causes, including damage to the spinal cord, immobility and the side effects of certain drugs, including several painkillers, or following changes to your diet.[6] If you are fatigued, you might feel that you do not have the energy to make a high-fibre meal or make sufficient drinks to keep you hydrated.

Most people need to drink the equivalent of between six and eight glasses of water a day, but this varies from person to person. You should drink enough fluid so that you're not thirsty for a long time. You will need to drink more when exercising and during hot weather. If your urine is clear or pale yellow, you're probably well hydrated. Dark, strong-smelling urine can be a sign of dehydration. As mentioned above, cloudy urine may be a sign of a urinary tract infection.

If you think you have diarrhoea or constipation, record how many times you pass a bowel movement and its consistency. You could keep a diary for a few days using the Bristol Stool Chart (<www.sthk.nhs.uk/library/documents/stoolchart.pdf>), which is widely used by doctors and nurses; then go and see your GP or MS team. If it is obvious that you have constipation or diarrhoea, see your GP and MS team as soon as possible.

Tips to tackle constipation

Do not take laxatives unless a healthcare professional tells you to. Instead, try the suggestions given below.

- Dehydration can make stools harder. Some people find that not drinking alcohol, coffee, tea and grapefruit juices, which can make you urinate more than plain water, helps avoid dehydration.
- Bland foods – such as rice, banana and apples – and eating more fibre may help avoid constipation.
- Try to take regular exercise, ideally for at least 30 minutes a day.
- Try to have regular bowel movements. You may find defecating after breakfast easier, when the bowel's contractions tend to be strongest. Try to go the toilet at the same time each day.

Tips to help bowel incontinence

If you develop incontinence of your faeces, you should tell your GP or MS team as soon as possible.[3] In the meantime, the following tips may help.

- Avoid caffeine, alcohol, fruit juices and smoothies.
- Avoid high-fibre, fatty, greasy and spicy foods.
- Try plain food (such as bananas, white bread, white fish, chicken or turkey).
- Eat small, frequent meals.
- Eat foods rich in pectin, which is the natural gelling agent found in ripe fruit that is used to make jams and jellies. Eating less fibre and more pectin-rich foods helps build your stools' consistency (Table 4).
- Diarrhoea can mean that you lose large amounts of a mineral called potassium, which muscles need to work properly.

Table 4 Foods rich in pectin, potassium or both

Foods rich in pectin
Apples, peeled or as sauce, without spices
Asparagus tips
Avocados
Bananas
Beets
Plain pasta
Potatoes, baked without skin
White bread
White rice
Foods rich in potassium
Apricot nectar
Asparagus tips
Avocados
Bananas
Fish
Peach nectar
Potatoes, boiled or mashed without skin

Potassium is also essential for normal nerve conduction. As a result, losing large amounts of potassium can leave you feeling weak and fatigued, so eat foods high in potassium to replace what you have lost (Table 4).

- If you experience diarrhoea, drink at least 2–3 litres a day, as diarrhoea can lead rapidly to dehydration.
- Try eating foods at room temperature: cold and hot foods tend to stimulate the gut.

Good hygiene is very important if you develop diarrhoea. Clean yourself carefully after each bowel movement. Use soft wipes and pat rather than rub the area around the anus. You could apply a barrier cream or ointment to protect this delicate area. Ask a pharmacist, GP or MS team if you are unsure about which barrier product to use or how to apply the cream or ointment.

Motor and balance difficulties

MS can cause one or more 'motor problems', such as weakness, tremor (uncontrolled shaking), poor dexterity and discomfort. Some people with MS find that walking feels as if they were floating, moving through water or snow, or stepping on eggs. These sensations seem to arise when MS damages the nerves that carry signals from our senses in the body to the brain.[13]

Other people develop weakness in a limb. The effect may be that some people drag one of their legs when they walk or find walking upstairs hard. Others need to sit down to perform everyday tasks such as peeling vegetables or ironing.[13]

Most people with MS find that, over time, walking becomes increasingly difficult and they eventually need a cane, wheelchair or other aid. However, two-thirds of people with MS can walk reasonably well for at least 15 years and may, at first, need aids only during relapses. Mobility difficulties that arise during a relapse may improve as you recover. Nevertheless, many people with MS still experience motor and balance difficulties between relapses.[3, 13]

The effects of MS on mobility vary widely both from person to person and in the same person, for example, depending on the severity of the relapse. Each person's goals also differ. You will probably see specialists in rehabilitation and physiotherapists with expertise in MS and they can devise an individualized programme to help you meet, as far as possible, your goals. So, as mentioned above, the following is for general guidance only.

Balance and gait issues

About three-quarters of people with MS experience difficulties with their balance, which can emerge early in the course of the disease.[13] According to NICE, 17 out of 20 (85 per cent) people with MS report that changes in the pattern of limb movement (gait) is one of their main difficulties. Once again, people with progressive MS tend to experience more severe balance difficulties than those with RRMS.[2] Balance and gait difficulties can emerge in several ways. Some people with MS find that their knees give way. Some people find they are prone to tripping. Others move as if they were drunk.[13]

Two underlying factors seem to contribute to balance difficulties in MS.[13, 19]

- Damage to the areas of the brain that control movement. For instance, damage to the pathways that connect the brain and the inner ear can cause vertigo, dizziness and difficulties with balance.
- Some MS symptoms, such as weakness, tremor, fatigue, numbness, problems with vision, fatigue, spasticity and ataxia (poor coordination). Muscle weakness, for example, can arise from damage to the nerve pathways or because the person uses the limb less. Tackling other symptoms of MS that influence balance often helps.

The benefits of physiotherapy

Physiotherapy seems to be especially effective in people with MS who develop mild-to-moderate difficulties with balance. Your physiotherapist can also help you devise an exercise programme that you should try to stick to after the formal therapy ends. So, if you feel that you sway when you stand upright or feel less stable when you move, it is worth mentioning this to your MS team. There are several approaches, including those given below.

- Some physiotherapy techniques 'teach' other parts of the brain to compensate for, or take over from, the damaged pathway –

so-called motor learning. (As mentioned on page 12, part of the brain called the cerebellum is important in motor learning.) Focusing physiotherapy on a specific task seems to encourage the brain to bypass the damaged area. This approach seems to be most effective in early or mild MS, but motor learning remains possible even in severe MS.[2]

- Exercises such as rocking, swinging, spinning, sitting on a beach ball, balance boards linked to a computer (a bit like a video game) and using a Swiss ball can help improve balance.[19]
- Using a treadmill or robot-assisted training can modestly improve gait even in people with severe MS. Computer-controlled automated devices that move a limb – essentially robots – can respond as the individual's needs change.
- A person with MS in a wheelchair may be able to learn new ways of self-care and domestic tasks, which helps maintain their independence.[2] The improvement is likely to be only partial, especially in advanced or more severe MS, and in older people.

Falls

Not surprisingly, people with MS who develop difficulties with balance and gait are especially prone to falls. Indeed, at least half of people with MS and poor balance fall over the following 6 months. Between 3 in every 10 and almost a half (29 to 49 per cent) of people with MS experience recurrent falls.[2] The risk of falls increases as the MS progresses. People with progressive MS are twice as likely to fall as those with RRMS.[2]

Falls increase the risk of a broken bone, especially as osteoporosis (which causes brittle bones) is particularly common in people with MS. In addition, people with MS are about twice as likely to injure themselves when they fall, compared with healthy people. Not surprisingly, a fear of falling can undermine confidence and independence as well as their ability to take part in the activities of daily life,[51] which is often not fully appreciated by families, friends and colleagues – something I've discovered after falling badly a couple of times due to arthritis. You may need to explain the effect on your confidence and independence to your family, friends and colleagues.

Reducing the risk of falls

How can you reduce the risks of falls?

- Occupational therapists can suggest adaptations to your home and workplace that make getting around safer and easier, such as ramps, handrails and grab bars.
- Badly fitting or inappropriate footwear, rushing and cognitive difficulties can all increase the likelihood of falls. A person with the latter may, for example, fall after taking unnecessary risks.
- If you are buying carpet, get one with a short pile. People with a cane, walker or wheelchair can find that longer carpet piles hinder their movement.
- Tuck extension cables and leads away.
- Ensure there is good lighting inside and outside the house.
- Stick down loose carpets and mats.
- Try to limit clutter, which can be a trip hazard as well as a distraction.
- Have non-slip surfaces in showers and baths.

Assistive technologies

Assistive technologies, such as the following, can help with specific difficulties.[19]

- A toe or finger spreader can relax tightness in the feet and hands, respectively.
- Braces for the wrist, foot and hand can maintain a natural position, which can prevent limitations of movement and deformities, as well as reducing the load on other joints. Your knee can come under considerable pressure if spasticity affects your ankle, for instance. Stress on joints, such as those produced by walking difficulties, can also cause considerable pain and may lead to arthritis.
- A neck brace may reduce tremors in the head, neck and upper torso.
- A forearm crutch provides greater stability than a cane and does not need as much upper body strength.
- A wheelchair or motorized scooter can help preserve your independence.

A therapist can help you choose the approach that best keeps you mobile.

Sticks, walkers and other assistive devices can aid mobility and help you remain independent. You're not 'giving in' to MS by using canes and other assistive technologies. I've been using a cane for the last couple of years, but for arthritis rather than MS. I've found that using a cane helps reduce the risk and fear of falls and stumbles, while increasing my confidence. Indeed, assistive technologies can help you overcome any limitations imposed by MS and help you take part in daily activities.[19] However, you will need professional help – even for a simple aid such as a cane, which needs to be measured properly. Indeed, I'm 6 foot 5, and my cane needed to be specially made.

Weakness

Up to 70 per cent of people with MS experience muscular weakness, most commonly in the legs and feet. Some of those with advanced MS experience weakness in the arms and hands, trunk and muscles you use to breathe. Not surprisingly, muscular weakness can affect movement, balance and the ability to perform normal activities.[2]

Weakness among people with MS typically arises from interruptions in the transmission of signals to the muscle because of demyelination in the spinal cord and, less commonly, the brain. However, weakness can have several other origins. Your MS team will work with you to identify the cause of the weakness, which can influence management.[19]

Building strength

Resistance training – such as using weight machines, free weights, a stationary bike that allows you to move the handlebar, a rowing machine or resistance bands – can help build muscular strength. You could also try, for example, cycling, swimming and exercises in water (such as aqua-aerobics).[2] Your physiotherapist can help you decide which works for you.

Strength training may help if weakness arises mainly in your muscles, but follow the therapists' advice. This is because exercising until you are fatigued can exacerbate weakness rather than boosting strength. If weakness arises from demyelination, lifting and weight training may make matters worse.[19] You could also try doing some of the things suggested below.

- Tackling the underlying cause may help if weakness arises from fatigue or spasticity.
- Save your strength for practical and enjoyable activities by planning your time carefully (page 59). Try performing difficult or physically demanding activities before easier ones.[19]
- Ask for help with finding the right assistive technologies.[19]
- When MS affects muscles in the feet, your toes may touch the ground before your heel, which can disrupt your balance,[19] so wear properly fitted shoes with, if necessary, inserts.[19] Your MS team can help.

Ataxia

At least 4 in every 5 people with MS develop ataxia (poor coordination) at some point.[2] In other words, you may seem clumsy. You may find putting make-up on or using tools more difficult. You may drop things or have more accidents.[13]

Ataxia often proves difficult to manage. Some drugs, surgical procedures and rehabilitation help some people. You might also be able to learn some strategies that at least partly compensate, such as those given below.[2]

- You may be able to break down a more complex movement into stages. Ask your physiotherapist or MS team if you need help with this.
- Your physiotherapist or MS team may be able to help you use visual cues to help with walking speed and stride length.
- Ask your physiotherapist, MS team or patient group if any aids might help. For instance, garments made of Lycra may improve the stability and function of your trunk.
- Biofeedback (page 119) using virtual reality or a machine that measures a muscle's electrical activity can help ataxia. Computer games that require balance and coordination help some people with MS improve their balance and avoid falls.[2]

If you feel that you are clumsier than before, it is worth telling your MS team or GP.

Spasticity and spasms

A balance of nerve signals controls each muscle. One set of nerve signals tells your muscles to contract; another tells your muscles to relax. The balance between the two allows you to make the most delicate fine movements – such as threading a needle – or the large coordinated actions throughout your body needed when, for instance, you run and catch a ball, or ride a bike. MS can disrupt this fine balance. For example:

- if MS interrupts the signals telling muscles to contract, your limbs may become limp and floppy;
- if MS disrupts the signals telling muscles to relax, you may develop stiffness and involuntary muscle spasms (a spasm is a sudden stiffening of a muscle) and, during a spasm, a limb may fly outwards or jerk towards your body.

A common difficulty

Between 6 and 9 in every 10 (60 to 90 per cent) people with MS develop spasticity.[2] Some individuals with MS-related spasticity develop a mild feeling of tightness and stiffness in the arms or, especially, the legs, which may make walking difficult. In severe cases, the tightness affects muscles throughout the body and may confine the person to bed or a wheelchair. Spasticity can reduce the joints' range of movement and contribute to pain and pressure sores. Not surprisingly, spasticity can reduce quality of life and the person's ability to take part in social activities.[2]

People with MS usually find that spasticity predominately affects the muscles they use to stay upright and walk around, so you might

Describing spasticity

Neurologists may use several terms to describe the pattern of spasticity, including:

- **hemiparesis**   partial paralysis or weakness of the entire left or right side of the body;
- **paraparesis**   partial paralysis or weakness of the lower limbs;
- **quadriparesis**   partial paralysis or weakness of all four limbs;
- **single-limb spasticity.**[6]

expend a lot more energy than usual on the ordinary activities of everyday life. Alleviating spasticity can reduce fatigue.[19]

If not adequately treated, severe spasticity can mean that muscles remain stiff and tight for a long time. These 'contractures' can pull joints into abnormal positions or prevent the normal range of motion. Contractures tend to be painful, can become permanent and can lead to muscle shortening.

Physiotherapy for spasticity

Several MS symptoms can exacerbate spasticity, including constipation, pain, fatigue, stress, heat, poorly fitting mobility aids, bad posture, pressure sores, and urinary tract and other infections. Treating these can improve spasticity.[19]

Physiotherapy and exercise seem to alleviate spasticity, improve quality of life and enhance gait. In addition, physiotherapy and exercise may reduce the risk of osteoporosis and heart disease.[6] Before considering a treatment for spasticity, you and your MS team should agree on the aim of treatment. Is the main goal to improve, for example, seating posture? Or is it to reduce painful spasms?[6]

Physiotherapy and exercise often help manage muscle stiffness, even if you also receive an anti-spasticity medicine (see below). As your symptoms, disabilities and goals are unique to you, the physiotherapist will fully evaluate how well you can move and develop an individualized programme. In addition, according to some studies, exercise may delay the progression of MS by reducing inflammation and encouraging repair of damaged nerves.[2]

Typically, a therapist may suggest an exercise programme, including, for example, the types of exercise given below.

- Aerobic exercise.
- Aqua-aerobics The buoyancy of water may reduce the amount of energy a person with MS expends – which helps with fatigue – while enhancing the efficient use of many muscles. Your physiotherapist can help develop a programme that allows the body to move through as much a range as possible, while supported by the water.[19]
- Specific exercises to improve posture and balance.
- Passive stretching A physiotherapist, another healthcare professional or a carer slowly and gently moves the joint into a

position that stretches the spastic muscle. You and your helper hold the position for about a minute and then slowly relax the muscle, which helps release the tension.

- **Muscle strengthening** (see above).
- **Range of motion exercises**, which move the joint through the full range of movements.[6] The stretch isn't held for any specific time. As you might need to work on several joints, you might need to be patient with your progress.[19]
- **Relaxation techniques**, such as PMR, deep breathing and imagery can help alleviate spasticity.[19] However, always check with your MS team or physiotherapist before you begin any additional therapy. PMR (page 95) may not be suitable for some people with muscular or joint problems, for example.

Baclofen and gabapentin

Doctors can prescribe several medicines that may help alleviate spasticity. NICE suggests that people with MS should manage their symptoms of spasticity by adjusting doses of drugs within limits agreed with their team. For example, NICE suggests trying baclofen or gabapentin depending on other health issues, any other medicines that you are taking and your preferences. If baclofen does not work adequately, you can switch to gabapentin and vice versa. Sometimes they are given together.

Baclofen relaxes muscles. The doctor will gradually increase the dose, which helps find the right balance, but some people still develop excessive weakness. Sometimes people lose tone in their trunk and sitting becomes difficult. In addition, increased muscle tone can act as a 'splint' for the legs, so some people taking baclofen find that their disability increases. Baclofen can also cause several other side effects, including dizziness, drowsiness, increased need to pass urine, headache and, rarely, seizures.[6]

Gabapentin, which you also take by mouth, may be effective if you also experience central neuropathic pain or painful spams.[6] However, side effects include: an increased risk of infection; feeling drowsy or dizzy; lack of coordination; feeling tired; changes in appetite or mood; confusion and difficulty with thinking; and sensations such as pins and needles. Clearly, some of these overlap with MS, which can complicate diagnosis of the underlying cause.

Doctors may offer people with severe spasticity intrathecal baclofen, which is pumped through a small tube directly into the CSF (page 39). The pump is implanted in the abdomen and needs to be refilled from time to time. As baclofen is administered directly into the spinal canal, the person receives very low doses, which reduces the risk of side effects. However, some people report nausea, drowsiness, urinary retention and dangerously low blood pressure (severe hypotension). Very rarely, the pump can fail, which can cause severe 'rebound' spasticity, confusion, seizures and, occasionally, organ failure.[6]

A word of warning

Many drugs used to treat spasticity can cause sedation or affect coordination. If you experience drowsiness or your coordination suffers, do not drive, operate machinery or take part in any activity that could prove hazardous.[6]

Other medicines

Several other medicines can help with spasticity, including those listed below.

- **Tizanidine** seems to be, in general, as effective as baclofen, and many people find that they are less likely to suffer side effects. About 1 in 20 people who take tizanidine show changes in levels of liver enzymes,[6] which may indicate liver damage.
- **Dantrolene** acts directly on muscles and may avoid some CNS side effects, such as sedation and poor coordination. Dantrolene can cause gastrointestinal problems, liver toxicity and breathing difficulties, however.[6] NICE suggests taking tizanidine or dantrolene if gabapentin or baclofen do not provide adequate relief.
- **Benzodiazepines** can cause sedation and muscle weakness. The doses are similar to those used to treat anxiety, which may help address two problems at once.[6] Benzodiazepines can cause addiction and tend to be used when other drugs fail.
- **Botulinum toxin injection** can relieve small areas of spasticity for about three months.[6]
- **Surgery** can occasionally alleviate resistant cases of spasticity.[6]
- **Nabiximols** (also called **Sativex**), which is derived from cannabis

(page 118), is effective for moderate to severe spasticity that has shown an inadequate response to other treatments or when these have produced unacceptable side effects. Nabiximols, which you spray into your mouth, can cause side effects, including dizziness, drowsiness, diarrhoea, fatigue, nausea, headache and a dry mouth. Nabiximols is not recommended for pregnant women or people with a history of psychotic illness.[6] Some studies associate schizophrenia with cannabis use, especially when marijuana is used in adolescence. Unlike medical marijuana (page 118), nabiximols is legal if prescribed by a doctor.

Tremor

Tremor (uncontrolled shaking) in people with MS often seems to follow damage to a part of the brain called the thalamus.[19] The thalamus carries sensory and motor signals to the cerebral cortex – the thin outer layer of the brain that processes information. Once again, tremors are typically more common in people with progressive MS than RRMS.

Types of tremor

Doctors recognize several types of tremor.

- **Action tremors** occur when you want to voluntarily contract a muscle or support part of your body against gravity, such as keeping your arm outstretched.
- **Intention tremors**, as the name suggests, arise when you want to perform a certain movement, such as touching your nose with your finger.
- **Rest tremors** occur while you are resting in bed or a chair and are not deliberately contracting a muscle.

Managing tremor can prove difficult, and severe cases may need surgery. Nevertheless, a range of drugs and physiotherapy can help.[6] For example, a physiotherapist or occupational therapist can also help you compensate, especially if the tremor affects the limbs, and provide as much stability as possible.[19] The approaches given below, for example, can be used.

- **Patterning** Repeating a movement eventually means it becomes automatic. You had to repeatedly perform a sequence of movements when you learnt to catch a ball, ride a bike or walk, for example. Now you can repeat the pattern without thinking. A therapist can use the same principle to lay down a new pattern of movement in your brain. The therapist will guide the movement until it becomes automatic. Once you make the movement automatically, you may then perform the action against mild resistance, which helps build endurance.[19]

- **Immobilization** A brace fixes the joint in position. This dampens the tremor and, when used for the ankle and foot, can provide a stable base for moving and standing. Braces can also help keep the body in a position that helps with specific tasks, such as writing or eating. You can remove the brace when you have finished the task.[19]
- **Weighting** Adding weights to parts of the body (such as the hand, wrist, foot or ankle) or to an object (such as a kitchen utensil, pen, cane or walker) can enhance control. Essentially, adding a weight 'recruits' support from other muscles around the area weakened by the MS. This stabilizes the tremor and provides more sensory feedback to the brain.[19] This, in turn, allows you to better control your movements.
- **Adjusting your posture** Physiotherapists may suggest adjustments, such as trying to keep your arms close to your body when performing tasks.[19]
- **Thalamotomy** This operation may be suggested by your MS team if the above approaches fail. A thalamotomy destroys damaged parts of the thalamus. This may alleviate tremor that does not respond to other approaches.[19]

Speech difficulties

During the nineteenth century, several doctors – most famously Pierre Paul Broca, professor of anatomy at the University of Paris – found that damage to a small part of the brain robbed the person of the power of speech. Broca's area, usually on the left side of the brain, helps control speech and language. A complex and complicated network of nerves connects the areas of the brain that help us understand language and control speech to the voice box and lungs.

Your speech patterns may change if MS damages one of these pathways. For example, people with MS often have a flatter intonation and may slur certain words. Tremors of the lips, tongue or jaw can also make speech difficult.[3, 19] Speech may slow, especially when you are tired. As MS progresses, speech may become increasingly slurred, jerky, garbled or muddled.[13]

Speech therapists can help improve the rhythm and clarity of your speech. A speech therapist can, for example, help you adjust your rate of speaking, your phrasing and the ways you form words.[3, 19] In addition, a growing range of adaptations aid communication: think of Stephen Hawking's eloquence despite his profound disability.

Swallowing difficulties

A healthy person swallows about 600 times a day, usually when eating or drinking and about 50 times while asleep.[52] Each swallow results from a complex, coordinated sequence of movements that transport food and drink from the mouth through the pharynx, down the oesophagus and into the stomach.[52] MS that affects one of these stages in this pathway can lead to difficulties swallowing (dysphagia). In addition, aspiration – breathing food, saliva, liquids or vomit into the lungs – encourages the growth of bacteria, leading to pneumonia (infection of the lungs or large airways). Carers and people with MS should therefore watch for signs that might indicate dysphagia, such as:

- a feeling that the food 'becomes stuck' or is 'held up';
- coughing or choking;
- difficulty controlling food in the mouth;
- gurgling after swallowing;
- nasal regurgitation;
- difficulties swallowing;
- a 'wet voice' after swallowing.

Helping with swallowing difficulties

A speech therapist or dietitian can help by, for example, teaching alternative swallowing manoeuvres, suggesting exercises to improve swallowing and helping you find the best position in which to eat.

Tucking the chin in, for example, helps some people swallow. The advice given below might also help.

- Do not try to talk when you eat.
- Chew small portions well.
- Swallow more than once a bite.
- Swallow each mouthful before eating or drinking any more.
- Take your time; mealtimes should be relaxed and quiet.
- Try eating smaller meals more frequently, rather than three larger meals a day.
- Do not mix food and drink in the same mouthful.

If you develop swallowing issues, it is all too easy to become dehydrated and miss out on essential nutrients and the energy you need. This could make your fatigue and weakness worse. Your dietitian may suggest shakes, drinks and other foods that are easy to swallow and can help make up any nutritional shortfall.

You should think of these 'oral nutritional supplements' as being as much a part of your treatment as your medicines, so take them as the dietitian suggests and make sure that your GP continues to prescribe what the dietitian has advocated. A simple protein shake, which is the usual supplement prescribed by doctors, is ideal for some people, but it isn't for everyone. There is now a very wide range of supplements, so you should be able to find one that suits you and meets your nutritional needs. You can ask your MS team or GP to refer you to a dietitian with specific knowledge of helping people with MS.

6

The mental and emotional burden

Living under the shadow cast by MS can be intensely stressful even before you are 'officially' diagnosed. As we have seen, neurologists won't diagnose MS based on a single event, so you may need to wait months or even years before MS can be 'officially' diagnosed. And some people experience the clinically isolated syndrome and then never have other problem. This waiting and uncertainty can place an incredible strain on people with suspected MS and their families.

Once you've received the news that you have MS, you will need to adjust. You may need to readjust when you experience a relapse – and readjust again if you develop progressive MS. Your family may also go through similar adjustments. All this means that you might need to deal with considerable stress – on top of the day-to-day hassles we all face.

Ironically, however, that stress can trigger relapses.[6] MS also increases the risk of developing depression, anxiety and other psychological problems, so in this chapter we will look at some things you can do that might help you cope with the mental and emotional burden imposed by MS. If you ever feel you cannot cope or feel suicidal, seek help and support from your GP or MS team urgently (page 82).

Poor adaptation

Not surprisingly, some people find it hard to adapt mentally and emotionally to life with MS. Some people even deny that they have MS. Denial allows us to avoid accepting the reality of our situation – even when faced with overwhelming evidence. The classic example is drug addicts, gamblers and alcoholics, who minimize or deny the harm that they are doing to themselves and others. Similarly, a person with MS who is in denial may not want to hear about the disease or meet fellow sufferers. They may try to prove to doctors, the world and themselves that they do not have MS.[13]

Obviously, minimizing the impact – so that MS does not dominate your life – can help you cope. Denial, however, may mean you do not engage with conventional treatments, lifestyle changes and CAMs that could save you considerable suffering. People in denial may not adhere to treatment, for example, which can increase the risk of relapses and disability (page 50).

Isolation and anger

In other cases, people with MS become isolated. Taking some 'time out' can offer you the space you need to re-evaluate your life, goals, priorities and difficulties, and, in turn, develop a plan to cope. Many people, if they are lucky enough to be able to afford the trip, find a 'retreat' gives them the space they need. The less affluent of us could take a walk, sit in a café or just find some quiet time at home. However, taken to extremes, isolation can encourage apathy and depression. You could become cut off from friends, family, work and other social networks that can offer help and advice. If so, consider counselling or speaking to a helpline run by a MS support group.

Not surprisingly, being diagnosed with MS, or having the symptoms worsen, can leave some people feeling angry. Carers often bear the brunt of this anger. Don't bottle things up, though: expressing your emotions can be a valuable safety valve. Counsellors, spiritual advisers and patient groups can help you accept your anger and channel your emotions productively.

For example, some people – myself among them – find that listening to music is one of the best ways to relax, unwind and deal with illness and other causes of stress. Indeed, music produces measurable changes in the body, including reducing blood pressure and slowing heart rate and respiration.[53] Music therapy takes this a step further and uses singing, playing an instrument, drumming or listening to music to explore and cope with your feelings and emotions about your MS, its treatment and your prospects.

During art therapy, you use paint, clay, collage, sand or writing poetry or stories to express and understand your feelings. It works even if you are not artistic: the art is for your benefit, it is not going to appear at the National Gallery. Art therapy can release pent-up emotions, relieve stress, bolster your coping skills and help you identify issues that you need to resolve.[53]

When life becomes too much to bear

Many people find that living with MS involves enduring a series of crises. It is easy to feel isolated, overwhelmed and helpless, at least from time to time. Some people find the burden too much to bear: people with MS are about twice as likely to commit suicide as the rest of the population.[54] In many cases, suicide could have been avoided, so people with MS and their carers should watch for the warning signs that might suggest an increased risk of suicide.

The journey towards suicide typically develops in four stages.

- Initially, people think about suicide almost philosophically – so-called 'passive suicidal ideation'.
- People then move to 'active' suicidal ideation. They think about the suicide's impact on their family and friends, and consider how, when and where to kill themselves. This may include researching methods of suicide.
- They prepare to commit suicide. They may write a will, give away their possessions, write letters and place their affairs in order.
- Finally, they make the suicide attempt.[55]

If you find yourself at any of the four stages, seek help from a doctor, helpline, counsellor or your religious leader. However deep your suffering, remember that, as psychologist David Bresler remarks, 'suicide is a permanent solution to what might very well be a temporary problem' and 'if you act on these thoughts, you won't be around later on to change your mind'.[55]

If you feel you are suicidal or even feel that you are getting to the end of your tether, see your GP, go to A&E or phone a helpline, such as:

- Samaritans on 116 123
- Breathing Space on 0800 83 85 87
- HOPELineUK (aimed at people younger than 35 years of age and those concerned about a young person) on 0800 068 41 41.

You could also call the helplines run by MS support groups (page 125). Suicidal ideation, talk and attempts, as well as self-harm generally, are loud shouts for help. These helplines offer advice, support and comfort. They can help stop you making a decision you might not live long enough to regret.

Acceptance

Eventually, most people with MS reach a sense of peace as they learn how to cope with their emotions and feel in control again.[13] Some people and caregivers even find 'meaning' in their illness and use the MS as an impetus towards spiritual growth.

There are risks, however, even in acceptance. For example, acceptance is not the same as passivity. You need to be proactive to stick with your treatment, make plans and set goals to make the most of your life. The sooner you accept help and support, the better your quality of life will be.

A few words of advice for friends and relatives

If you are a relative or friend of a person with depression or another mental illness, always take suicide tendencies or talk seriously. Do not dismiss any of the following warning signs as attention-seeking[56] or 'just' a symptom of the MS:

- a period of agitation and then calm – this may reflect the torment of making the decision to commit suicide, and then a sense of peace once the decision is made;
- worsening of depression and hopelessness;
- changing a will;
- direct and indirect threats of suicide;
- discussing or preparing for suicide;
- giving away possessions, especially if valued or sentimental;
- isolation and loneliness;
- viewing websites about suicide.

Cognitive issues

According to NICE, between 2 in 5 and 7 in 10 (43 to 70 per cent) of people with MS develop difficulty with thinking, remembering and planning – so-called cognitive issues. These people with MS find they are not as 'mentally sharp' as they once were. They may experience difficulties concentrating. They may forget things,[3] including taking their medicines (page 51).

Cognitive problems may mean that it is hard for the person with MS to find and keep a job, manage their relationships or finances, take part in social activities or even complete everyday household tasks or continue to drive. Cognitive issues can also increase the strain on carers, undermine physical rehabilitation and contribute to the risk of falls.[8] People with MS and cognitive issues also seem to be more likely to develop psychiatric ailments, such as depression and anxiety.

Cognitive problems can emerge during a relapse, and, as you might expect, they worsen as MS progresses. Brain scans show that the networks of nerves responsible for cognition become increasingly disorganized. Unfortunately, disease-modifying therapies seem to have less of a benefit on cognitive problems than on physical disability.[2]

NICE notes, however, that the person with MS may not immediately recognize that they have cognitive difficulties or link these to their MS. In addition, NICE notes that anxiety, depression, difficulty sleeping and fatigue can cause or contribute to cognitive issues, and tackling these symptoms can enhance cognition. It is important, therefore, to mention even subtle cognitive changes to your MS team.

Give your memory a helping hand

Whatever the cause – stress or the MS – you can give your memory a helping hand.

- Try memory aids, such as making lists or using a diary, for things you need to remember.
- Fix a routine, which can also help counter fatigue.
- Practise your mental skills by craftwork, chess, board or card games and some computer games.
- Exercise – even stretching and balancing – seems to slow the decline in cognition.[3]

These are only a few examples. A neuropsychologist or occupational therapist can identify your particular pattern of cognitive difficulties and find tailored ways to help.

Depression: an unshakable sadness

Is it any wonder that a person who is diagnosed with a life-changing disease, such as MS, becomes depressed? Is it any wonder that a person with MS feels depressed as their MS progresses and they begin to lose bodily function? Is it any wonder that they feel anxious about being a burden to their families or friends?

That so many people with MS *do not* develop profound depression or anxiety amazes me. Nevertheless, about a quarter (25 per cent) of people with MS develop anxiety, while a third to half (34 per cent to 50 per cent) develop depression.[57] And unless you have suffered from depression or anxiety, it is difficult to appreciate just how devastating these can be.

In addition, people with MS are vulnerable to developing other psychiatric conditions, including bipolar disorder (previously called manic depression) and schizophrenia.[58] Furthermore, up to 1 in 10 people with MS show pseudobulbar affect – abnormal and inappropriate laughing and crying.[2] People with secondary progressive MS seem to be at particular risk of pseudobulbar affect,[2] which seems to emerge after damage to the parts of the brain that regulate emotions.

Not surprisingly, people with more severe physical disability tend to shoulder a heavier psychological burden than those with less marked problems. In a study of people with MS from the UK:

- in those with low levels of disability, almost two-fifths (38 per cent) experienced at least mild anxiety, and almost a fifth (17 per cent) experienced at least mild depression;
- among those with high levels of disability, more than two-thirds (67 per cent) and almost three-quarters (72 per cent) experienced anxiety and depression, respectively.[59]

The core symptoms of depression

Although the symptoms of depression differ from person to person, doctors recognize several core features. These are not unique to depression, and some, such as fatigue, can overlap with MS, which can complicate diagnosis. Nevertheless, the more symptoms in Table 5 you have, the more likely you are to have depression, especially if they persist and interfere with your day-to-day life. See your GP as soon as you can if you have little interest or take little pleasure in doing things you used to enjoy, or your feel down, depressed or hopeless for most of the day, every day for more than two weeks. See your doctor *urgently* if:

- you feel that life is unbearable;
- you are considering or taking steps toward suicide or self-harming (page 82);

Table 5 Examples of the core symptoms of depression

Examples of psychological symptoms of depression

Considering suicide, self-harm or taking steps towards suicide

Continuous low mood or sadness

Feeling anxious or worried

Feeling hopeless and helpless

Feeling irritable and intolerant of others

Feeling ridden with guilt, especially if the guilt is excessive or unjustified

Feeling tearful or crying

Lack of interest in things or activities, especially if these were once important or enjoyable

Lacking motivation

Low self-esteem

Procrastination (finding it difficult to make decisions)

Examples of physical symptoms of depression

Change in appetite or weight (usually decreased, but may increase)

Changes to the menstrual cycle

Constipation

Feeling lethargic (moving more slowly than usual)

Lack of energy

Loss of libido

Sleep disturbances, such as finding it hard to fall asleep at night for more than about half an hour or early-morning waking

Speaking more slowly or less than usual

Unexplained aches and pains

Examples of social symptoms of depression

Avoiding contact with friends and family

Avoiding social activities

Neglecting and not being interested in your hobbies and interests

Poor performance at work, such as poor concentration, lack of motivation and absenteeism

Problems in your home and family life

Source Adapted from NHS Choices

- you are unable to meet your work, social and family obligations;
- you hear voices in your head – which are usually critical or defamatory – or experience visual hallucinations (hallucinations can be symptoms of a very serious condition called psychotic depression).

When depression hurts the body

About two-thirds of people with depression develop physical (also called somatic) symptoms, including:[56, 60, 61]

- aches and pains: many people find that these aches and pains seem to be 'everywhere' rather than in a specific place, such as a muscle or joint;
- back pain, especially in the lower back;
- breathing difficulty or breathlessness;
- chest pains;
- digestive problems – nausea, diarrhoea or constipation – and stomach pain;
- dizziness, light-headedness or feelings of faintness;
- headaches;
- difficulty swallowing;
- tiredness, exhaustion and fatigue.

As this brief list shows, some somatic symptoms of depression overlap with those caused by MS. Keeping a note of which symptoms emerge, when and if there are any triggers can help determine the cause and, therefore, the most appropriate treatment.

Anxiety: prudence gone awry

Sometimes anxiety is prudent, producing physical, mental and behavioural changes that warn us of, and help us deal with, potential dangers, such as when we walk alone late at night, especially through an unfamiliar or disreputable area. However, if anxiety nags away at you, you should ask for help.

Anxiety disorders arise when our natural 'fear' reaction is out of proportion to the threat or is excessively prolonged. Phobias offer the best example: being terrified by a 15-centimetre (6-inch) Brazilian Wandering Spider in your supermarket bananas is prudent – they produce a deadly venom; being terrified by a barely visible money spider is a phobia.

Fight or flight

Anxiety increases mental alertness and heightens the acuity of your senses to help you detect danger early. Adrenaline and other chemicals flood your body. Your heart beat increases. You breathe more rapidly. You sweat. Blood flows from your skin and your intestines to your muscles. That's why we go pale when we are extremely stressed or frightened. Muscles surrounding the hair follicles tighten. That's why we get goose bumps. Our pupils dilate.

These changes are part of the 'fight-or-flight' response, which evolved to get us out of trouble quickly with the least possible damage. The fight-or-flight response was a lifesaver when our ancestors faced a rival tribe on the warpath or a hungry carnivorous animal. Unfortunately, the 'fight-or-flight' response does not distinguish between barbarian hordes and a pile of final demands, or between a ravenous sabre-toothed cat and life with MS.

When to seek help

You may find that your anxiety stems from a particular issue.

- Jot down everything that bothers you about your MS and your life generally, no matter how trivial. Try breaking big issues – such as living with MS – into smaller, specific difficulties, such as those that undermine your ability to take part in everyday activities or cause you discomfort.
- Use this list to home in on the issues that cause you the most distress. Try ranking each one on a scale of 0 to 10, where 1 is no distress and 10 is the most distress you have experienced or can imagine.
- See how your MS team and others can help you address the issue and, in turn, alleviate your anxiety. You could, for example, discuss a change in your treatment or additional support.
- Anxiety can arise if you do not fully understand something, such as getting the risk of treatment into perspective. Jot down your five biggest unanswered questions about MS and its treatment. Then talk to your MS team or call a support group helpline to clarify anything you don't understand.

Your needs, circumstances and treatments change over time, so even if you do not think you will use this technique now, try it if you find yourself feeling anxious, stressed or wound up in the future. Any chronic disease can overshadow your life, so you may find that many of the things that bother you have nothing to do with your MS.

In other cases, anxiety may be more generalized. In other words, you cannot tie the anxiety down to a particular cause. Answering 'Yes' to either of the following questions suggests that you may have 'generalized' anxiety.[62]

- During the past four weeks, have you been bothered by feeling worried, tense or anxious most of the time?
- Are you frequently tense, irritable and having trouble sleeping?

Treating anxiety and depression

Do not ignore anxiety or depression. Quite apart from the impact on your quality of life, people with MS and mental health issues may be less likely to follow their team's advice, may experience more severe symptoms and may be more likely to encounter problems with day-to-day activities and social life. On the other hand, increasing feelings of control and acceptance can lessen the psychological and emotional impact.[63] That's why CAMs can help: they enhance your sense of control.

Treatment of anxiety and depression is similar to that in people without MS. Often a talking treatment, such as CBT (see below), is more effective than drugs for anxiety or depression.[6]

Locus of control

Psychologists describe the extent to which you feel you control your life as your 'locus of control'. A strong internal locus of control means you tend to see yourself as in charge of your life. If you have a strong external locus of control, you see yourself as having little influence over your life. You feel that events – such as living with MS – control you. As a result, people with an external locus of control react worse to stress than those with an internal locus of control[64] and are especially prone to developing anxiety and depression. Talking therapies, CAMs and counselling can bolster your internal locus of control.

Support groups and services

In addition, many people with MS find that they benefit from taking part in support groups or local support services. The latter are often run by volunteers from a patient organization and offer practical and emotional support, including help to access additional services. Support groups allow you to share your experiences with others and find help with particular problems. Some people with MS are sceptical until they take part – and then realize the group's value. Your MS team or a patient organization can help you find a local group or support team.

There are also numerous online forums and social media groups. These can be useful when, for example, you're fatigued and want to save your energy for other things. They also allow naturally shy or geographically isolated people with MS to access additional advice and support.

Keep working

It's worth making an effort to keep and develop relationships with family and friends, and to stay in work for as long as possible. Working, assuming you are physically and mentally able, can help keep depression at bay and bolster the family finances. Going back to work after a relapse can be a sign that things are getting back to normal.

You should think about telling your employer and colleagues, even though many will have only a vague understanding of MS. In particular, employers and colleagues can find it hard to appreciate the impact of fatigue, pain and other less obvious symptoms. You might find that leaflets from MS support groups or pointing them towards a website helps. In some cases – such as if you drive for a living, you are in the armed forces or the MS could affect health and safety at work – you must tell your employer. Your MS team and support groups can help if you are unsure whether or not to tell your employer or mention your condition on a job application.

Unfortunately, about half of people with MS are unemployed. Many of these are simply unable to work, but, if you can, it's worth trying to stay in employment. (I don't, just to make it clear, support forcing people back to work by threatening benefit payments. You should work only if you are able to.)

You may need to ask your MS team or GP to treat any depression and anxiety, which can make returning to work more difficult. Telling your employer you have MS can help if you need some adaptations at work. You may also need to ask for flexibility in your working arrangements (if you feel fatigued or need treatment in hospital, for example). And, of course, you may need time off and to ease back into work if you experience a relapse.[3] You and your employer also have certain obligations under, at the time of writing, the Equality Act and the Disability Discrimination Act, so you could speak to a union rep, patient group or social worker about your rights. The MS Trust has an excellent summary of the current legislation.

Your MS team can put you in touch with a medical social worker or an occupational therapist who can help you remain in work. You can also think about changing your position within your company or getting another job to help you live with MS or progress your career. The UK National Careers Service and patient groups' helplines and websites can help you decide if this is right for you, and advise you on what you should disclose to a new employer.

Cognitive behavioural therapy

In 1976, the American psychiatrist Aaron Beck suggested that fear and anxiety arise when the person 'senses' danger and anticipates that they or a loved one could come to harm. Depression, Beck argued, arises from a feeling that you have lost something important forever. Beck suggested that you feel happy when you experience pleasure or expect a positive event.[65]

Beck believed that events do not *directly* cause anxiety, depression and other emotional problems. Rather, our interpretation of an event determines whether we develop anxiety, depression or another psychiatric condition. You view the same event in different ways depending on whether you are happy and relaxed or depressed and anxious. For instance, when you are anxious, you may interpret a minor ailment that has no connection to the demyelination as 'proof' that your MS is getting worse. When you are depressed, you may feel you have MS-related fatigue rather than the lassitude that is all too often the handmaiden of mood disorders. Negative emotions and expectations feed off each other, exacerbating depression or anxiety.

Beck's theory forms the foundation of CBT,[65] one of the most widely used talking therapies. CBT identifies feelings, thoughts and behaviours associated with your MS itself or that contribute to your anxiety or depression. Some of these feelings, thoughts and behaviours are appropriate and helpful. Sometimes extra support from your MS team can tackle some triggers for anxiety and depression or address an issue identified by CBT that is causing you distress.

Essentially, CBT replaces the remaining, counterproductive feelings, thoughts, behaviours and beliefs. CBT is not the same as positive thinking. Indeed, unrealistic positive thinking can become a form of denial (page 80). CBT is about striking a balance between optimism and pragmatism.

Your therapist may ask you to record negative thoughts and behaviours in a diary. You can then look at the evidence for and against each thought and behaviour. Finally, you can replace counterproductive ideas with more objective and rational approaches, which help you cope more effectively and efficiently as you live with MS. CBT usually uses explicit objectives, broken into manageable, short-term goals and supported by regular 'homework'.

How effective is CBT?

CBT and the other psychotherapies (talking therapies) are usually the treatment of choice for depression or anxiety in general as well as for people with MS. Increasingly, doctors prescribe antidepressants and anxiolytics only for severe depression or anxiety, often combined with psychotherapy, or when non-drug treatments do not offer sufficient relief. Indeed, CBT seems to be as effective as the antidepressant sertraline against depression in people with MS. CBT and other forms of psychotherapy help people with MS develop coping skills that tackle unhelpful thoughts, inappropriate emotions and counterproductive adjustments, such as denial.[66]

CBT may even reduce disease progression in people with MS.[63] According to one study, in the short term, CBT's disease-modifying effects are similar to those produced by some drugs.[63] As stress can affect the immune system, this is not perhaps surprising, but further studies are needed. It is important to never stop taking a prescribed drug – or reduce the dose – without speaking to your MS team first.

Mindfulness and meditation

Essentially, mindfulness and meditation encourage you to concentrate, non-judgementally and openly, on the present rather than worry about what might happen or ruminate on the past. Mindfulness and meditation allow you to take a step back from your anxiety, depression, stress and other emotions. As such, mindfulness and meditation seem to increase your ability to regulate your behaviour, thoughts and emotions, as well as improving the flexibility of your thinking and enhancing your attention. Some people report that mindfulness and meditation are a bit like waking up from life on automatic pilot.

Mindfulness-based training lasting between six and eight weeks seems to improve quality of life as well as some mental and physical symptoms in people with MS, such as balance, pain, depression, anxiety and fatigue. Indeed, the benefits of mindfulness seemed to last for at least six months. However, further studies are needed to fully understand the role of mindfulness-based interventions in MS care.[57, 63] Mindfulness encourages you to become more aware of your body and its response to internal and external stimuli.[67] However, people with MS may already be highly sensitive to mental and physical changes, so try not to become preoccupied with how you feel.

Mindfulness or meditation

Mindfulness-based training can take various forms. Typically, however, mindfulness includes mindful breathing (sitting and 'watching' the breath) and mindful movement – which might use elements of tai chi, qi gong or yoga. Mindfulness-based training can also include elements from CBT. Mindfulness generally emphasizes regular practice, which may mean investing, for example, 30 to 40 minutes a day.[63]

In many ways, mindfulness is similar to the early stages of the meditation techniques taught by Buddhism and some other Eastern religions and certain types of prayer, but stripped of the religious connotations. Indeed, meditation is not confined to sitting in the lotus position for hours chanting 'om' or another mantra: most people find it easier to be more aware while walking or moving. Tai chi, qi gong, yoga and rosary prayer are forms of meditation. Your vicar or spiritual adviser can offer advice about prayer.

Learning classical meditation or mindfulness can be difficult without face-to-face guidance; you could see if your local adult education centres hold courses. To get a taste of mindfulness or mediation, focus on a single object, idea, subject or sensation – such as the flow of your breath in and out of your mouth or nose. If you mind wanders off, bring it back to your focus. Try not to get annoyed if you find this difficult, especially as it is often much harder than it sounds. After a few minutes, stop and relax. As you practise every day, you will be able to gradually increase the time you remain focused.

Relaxation therapy

As a way to relax, there is nothing wrong with curling up with a good book or watching your favourite television programme or DVD. However, many of us, not just people with MS, need to take a more 'active' approach to relaxation. Indeed, relaxation therapy can improve quality of life for people with MS.[57] In one study, for example, almost 3 in 5 (57 per cent) people who used PMR reported that their pain intensity decreased by about a third or more (at least 30 per cent).[47] Relaxation techniques, such as breathing deeply, can prevent the hyperventilation and other manifestations of anxiety that some people experience with injectable MS drugs.[43]

The following tips should help you relax. You may need to adapt these if, for example, you want to meditate or practise yoga.

- Find time for your relaxation therapy every day. Many people find that the early morning is the best for 'active relaxation'. The house is quiet and you will be better able to focus and less likely to drop off to sleep than later at night.
- Sit in a comfortable chair that supports your back, or lie down. You may want to put cushions under your neck and knees. Take off your shoes, switch off bright lights and ensure the room is a comfortable temperature.
- Do not try to perform relaxation therapy on a full stomach. After a meal, blood diverts from your muscles to your stomach. Trying PMR on a full stomach can cause cramps. And relaxation can make you more aware of your body's functions so a full stomach can be a distraction.
- Shut your eyes and, if it helps, play some relaxing music and burn some aromatherapy oils (page 116). Some people, for example, find that lavender helps them relax.

Follow your relaxation regimen, such as guided imagery, meditation or PMR. A counsellor or meditation or mindfulness course can
help you integrate regular relaxation into your lifestyle.

Progressive muscular relaxation

To try progressive muscular relaxation (PMR), follow the steps given
below.

- Put your hands by your sides. You can stand, sit or lie down.
  Now clench your fists as hard as you can. Hold the fists tight for
  ten seconds.

Think about your breathing

One of the first things that a yoga, martial arts or meditation
teacher will probably tell you is that you are not breathing correctly.
Breathing correctly can produce marked physical and mental
changes. For example, changes in the number of breaths you take
can alter your heart rate by 12 to 15 beats per minute. As you
breathe more deeply, more oxygen reaches your blood and your
heart does not need to work as hard: the brain detects the increase
in oxygen, and nerves tell the heart that it does not need to pump as
hard.

This 'feedback' between mind and body means you do not feel
mentally stressed when your body is relaxed and vice versa. On the
other hand, breathlessness commonly triggers anxiety, and becoming
anxious unfortunately exacerbates breathlessness. Breathing too
quickly can also bring on anxiety.

Most of us breathe too shallowly, using the upper parts of our
lungs. Try putting one hand on your chest and the other on your
abdomen. Then breathe normally. Most people find that the hand on
their chest moves while the one on their abdomen remains relatively
still. To fill your lungs fully, try to make the hand on your abdomen
rise, while keeping the one on the chest as still as possible. Breathing
deeply and slowly without gasping helps relaxation.

You can try breathing as described below as a first aid for stress or
if you find you experience 'needle phobia'.

- Breathe in deeply through your nose for a count of four.
- Hold your breath for a count of seven.
- Breathe out for a count of eight.
- Repeat this a dozen times.

- Now slowly relax your fists and let your hands hang or rest on the floor loosely by your sides. Then shrug your shoulders as high as you can. Hold for ten seconds and then slowly relax.
- Now, while inhaling, gently arch your back. Hold this for ten seconds, making sure you breathe as slowly and rhythmically as you can. After the ten seconds, exhale as you relax.
- Repeat each exercise three times, slowly, gently and gradually.

Most PMR teachers advise mastering one muscle group at a time. It could take two or three months before you can tense and relax your entire body. Speak to your doctor before trying PMR if you have problems with your muscles, joints or bones, either because of your MS or from another ailment.

Sexual issues

MS can take its toll on relationships: as we have already seen, the divorce rate is twice that of the rest of the population when one person has MS.[3] Numerous factors contribute to the relationship issues that can affect people with MS. However, about half of people with MS experience sexual difficulties. The autoimmune attack can damage nerves that control erections and ejaculation in men as well as orgasm and genital sensations in both sexes. In addition, muscle weakness, fatigue, spasticity and loss of sensation can contribute to a loss of libido.[6]

The stress of living with a serious chronic disease as well as some of its obvious physical effects may also undermine libido in people with MS and their partners. Moreover, MS may affect the person's ability to work, which can contribute to financial difficulties – a common cause of libido-draining stress – or change the relationship's dynamic: for example, the carer may become the cared-for. Some people find the change reduces the partner's attractiveness. Other people, however, find the opportunities to help and be more intimate increase sexual desire. Nevertheless, partners should reassure people with MS that they remain attractive.

So overcome your embarrassment and speak to your MS team about problems with your sex life or with your relationship. They may be able to help in various ways.

- Some drugs can help with, for example, flaccid erections. (Never buy these over the Internet: they may be counterfeit, interact with other drugs you are taking or be dangerous if you have other health issues.)

- Sometimes a drug given to treat a symptom of MS can affect your sex life. Fortunately, there are usually alternatives.
- Counselling and simple changes can help if stress undermines your sex life.
- In addition to damage to the nerve pathways supplying the genitals, fatigue, depression, spasticity, anxiety and urinary difficulties can undermine libido. In many cases, treating the underlying cause can revitalize your sex life.

MS and pregnancy

MS typically emerges in relatively young people, so many women with MS want to have children. The good news is that pregnancy seems to reduce the likelihood of a relapse, probably because of alterations in hormones and changes to the immune system. These changes prevent the body from mounting an immune attack on the unborn baby, for example. The bad news, according to NICE, is that the rate of relapse may increase for 3 to 6 months after pregnancy. The risk then returns to normal. Being pregnant probably does not change the long-term course of your MS.

You will need to discuss treatment of MS during pregnancy with your team to reduce, as far as possible, the risk to the developing baby from the treatments. In many cases, the risks – if any – to the developing baby are not known. Treatment of MS during pregnancy is a particularly personal decision and one that needs careful discussion based on your circumstances and treatments, so we will not cover this here. However, you should have open discussions with your MS team as soon as you feel that you would like to have a baby or discover that you are pregnant. As mentioned above, you should always tell your MS team or doctor if you are, or think you might be, pregnant before taking steroids for a relapse.

Co-morbidities

People with MS often contend with more than symptoms arising from the nerve damage. They often have one or more other ailments (so-called comorbidities), such as heart disease, diabetes, bowel problems and so on. Indeed, the authors of a recent study noted that 'comorbidity is more common than expected in MS, even around the time of diagnosis'.[58] We have already seen that people with MS are especially prone to developing psychiatric conditions such as depression and anxiety, but it seems that people with MS are also prone to developing several physical problems.

There are several possible explanations for these links. For example, doctors may be more likely to diagnose a co-morbidity because of increased surveillance or simply because they see the person in clinic or the surgery more often. In addition, certain conditions may share risk factors. For instance, some of the same genes seem to contribute to MS and inflammatory bowel disease. Low levels of vitamin D seem to increase the likelihood of developing MS, heart disease, some cancers, diabetes and asthma.

Furthermore, many drugs for MS suppress the immune system. Although controlling the inflammation that damages the nerves helps to treat MS, suppressing the immune system may predispose to infections.[5, 58, 68] However, all drugs have side effects, and the benefits of the newer drugs outweigh the risks in most people with MS.

In addition, people with MS are at risk of developing secondary problems from their MS or its treatment. If you need a catheter, for instance, you may develop urinary tract infections. If your MS hinders your movement and ability to exercise, you might:[3]

- become overweight or obese, which may increase the risk of diabetes, heart disease and some cancers;
- develop pressure sores;
- be at risk of osteoporosis, caused by brittle bones.

In other words, watch out for any symptoms – do not dismiss them as part of your MS. Remember to take a list of medicines to each appointment with your MS team. They will need to know what you are taking – whether prescribed or bought from a shop or pharmacist, and any CAM – to avoid potentially serious interactions (page 49).

Carers: look after yourself

Caring for a person with MS can be, at times, tough, especially as relapses sometimes seem to strike without warning and the long-term outlook is often uncertain. Carers should try to remain as positive as possible and offer encouragement as well as practical and emotional support. However, carers need to avoid the temptation to do too much for the person with MS. You need to walk a tightrope between helping and allowing the person with MS to maximize their independence and, therefore, their self-esteem. The MS team can help you get the balance right.

Some carers need to balance a job or childcare with looking after a person with MS, which can cause considerable stress. Furthermore, your relationships can change fundamentally. Children or spouses may, for example, find themselves in a 'parental' role. Often the person who cared for the rest of the family now needs care themselves. The entire family may need time to adjust to the diagnosis of MS or the news that the disease is beginning to progress.

The person with MS may live overshadowed by stress and practical problems, be afraid of becoming disabled, and feel upset at not being able to take part in previously enjoyed activities. They may feel depressed, angry, guilty and bad-tempered, which, as mentioned above, can place a considerable strain on relationships.

To look after your partner, you need to look after yourself. Try to sleep or unwind while your partner is resting, and get a good night's sleep – the tips on page 61 may help carers too. You should follow any advice offered by the MS team about the person's activity. You may feel you want to do more than this. However, your good intentions could place an unnecessary burden on your shoulders and undermine your partner's independence and self-confidence. Make sure you have time to yourself: you need to recharge your batteries. Helping yourself helps you help the person with MS.

You may need to be honest with yourself. Partners of people with MS often feel angry, guilty and resentful and other family members may feel they do not receive sufficient attention. Don't bottle these feelings up. Concealing or repressing your emotional pain and stress (or, indeed, bottling things up) can erode closeness in relationships, so think and talk about your feelings with your partner, friends and family or a counsellor. Carers Direct is a national information, advice and support service for carers in England (<www.nhs.uk/carersdirect>, 0300 123 1053).

7

Diet and MS

As we have seen, doctors and researchers have made important strides in understanding the biology of MS, although many current treatments can produce unacceptable side effects or have other limitations. As a result, people with MS often try unproven treatments, lifestyle changes, CAMs, such as acupuncture, reflexology and hypnosis,[6] and sometimes fundamental changes to their diet.

The link between diet and MS is complex. Over the years, researchers have suggested that several elements in the diet – including vitamins A and D, salt and omega-3 polyunsaturated fatty acids (PUFAs) – can affect the immune system and, potentially at least, influence MS risk.[18] To take just one example, published as I was writing this book, researchers reported that, compared with people who did not drink coffee, the risk of MS was about a third (30 to 31 per cent) less common in those who drank more than about three mugs (900 to 948 ml) of coffee daily.[69]

To complicate matters further, CAM practitioners have suggested a variety of foods and supplements that they claim may alleviate MS. Some, but not all, of these dietary changes overlap with the scientific data. CAM practitioners may suggest, for example, antioxidants, low-carbohydrate diets, alfalfa sprouts, wheatgerm and omega-3 PUFAs. The conventional medical view is that little evidence suggests these foods and supplements are effective in MS – although there are relatively few studies.[3] However, a diet rich in antioxidants, low in carbohydrate and that contains alfalfa sprouts, wheatgerm and omega-3 PUFAs is undoubtedly healthy and would probably reduce the risk of other diseases, including heart disease, stroke and some cancers.

If you want to follow a specific diet for MS, therefore, learn all you can about it and make sure you will still get all the energy and nutrients you need. It is a good idea to speak to your MS team – and ideally a dietitian – before you make big changes to your diet.

The microbiome

The human body is home to some 100 trillion bacteria[70] as well as a range of fungi, viruses and other organisms. Biologists call this the 'microbiota' or 'microbiome'. The lower gut alone is home to more than 30,000 strains of bacteria. By way of contrast, the most generous estimate suggests that undisturbed tropical rainforest is home to 15,000 species.[70] Bacteria in the gastrointestinal tract break down foods that we cannot otherwise digest. The bacteria in our guts also boost the energy released from our diets by about 10 per cent, make vitamin K (which is essential for normal blood clotting), shape our immune responses and reduce the risk of several diseases, including colorectal cancer and obesity.[71-74]

Increasing evidence suggests that the composition of bacteria in the gut may influence the risk of MS.[75-78] Clinical studies are, therefore, underway to see if altering the balance helps in MS,[78] so it is worth keeping an eye on the patient group websites. In the meantime, there are numerous probiotic supplements and drinks available from supermarkets and health food shops that may help you restore a more balanced gut flora. Although there is, as yet, little direct evidence that these help MS, they may help bolster health more generally. If you want to take one of the more expensive and higher dose supplements than you buy at the supermarket, it is worth checking with the MS team first.

Omega-3 PUFAs

Life inside the Arctic Circle is tough. Few plants survive, so the traditional diet of first nation Arctic people consists of fish and animals that, in turn, eat marine life, such as seals and whales. Yet those who eat the traditional meat-based diet seem to be less likely to develop several diseases – including diabetes, heart disease, arthritis and asthma – than people in 'industrialized' countries. These are all diseases in which inflammation has an important role.

Fish and animals that survive on marine life are rich in omega-3 PUFAs, which seems to account for much of the benefit offered by the Arctic diet. For example, omega-3 PUFAS, among their other actions:

- reduce blood pressure and protect the heart and blood vessels from disease;

- are important for memory, intellectual performance and healthy vision – all of which can take a change for the worse in people with MS;
- may protect against and treat depression, which is common in MS;
- help reduce joint pain and stiffness – MS and rehabilitation can place extra stresses and strains on your joints (I take cod liver capsules for osteoarthritis and I'm convinced that they are one of the few things that really help);
- dampen general inflammation.

Fish and shellfish are good sources of many other nutrients such as vitamins A and D, iodine, calcium and selenium, as well as being an excellent source of protein. Everyone should, therefore, try to eat two portions of fish a week, one of which should be oily fish. White fish

Table 6 Examples of fish and seafood high in omega-3 fatty acids

Anchovy

Black cod (sablefish)

Crab (fresh)

Dogfish (rock salmon)

Halibut

Herring

Kippers

Mackerel

Mussels

Oysters

Pilchards

Rainbow trout

Salmon

Sardines

Shark and marlin

Sprats

Swordfish

Tuna (especially bluefin)

Whitebait

Source Adapted from the University of Michigan and the British Dietetic Association (such as cod, haddock, plaice, Dover sole) contain omega-3 PUFAs, but it is not as good a source of these as the oily fish listed in Table 6.

Omega-3 PUFA levels are highest in fresh fish. If you are eating canned fish, check the label to make sure processing has not depleted the omega-3 PUFAs. I believe that it is worth trying to check that fish comes from sustainable stocks (<www.goodfishguide.org> or look for a label on the packaging showing that it has Marine Stewardship Council certification). If at first you do not like the taste of oily fish, do not give up without trying some different fish and a few recipes. Fish does not have to be battered, rolled in breadcrumbs or served with a dollop of ketchup or tartare sauce. There are plenty of suggestions on the internet (such as at <www. thefishsociety.co.uk>) and in cookbooks. For an island nation, our tastes in fish are remarkably conservative.

Mercury in fish

As we saw, mercury in fish was an important link in the chain leading to the tragic industrial accidents in Japan (page 21). According to the Food Standards Authority, the amount of mercury in food in the UK is not enough to harm most people. Nevertheless, pregnant women should not eat more than two tuna steaks (each about 140 g cooked or 170 g raw) or four medium-sized cans of tuna a week (each about 140 g when drained). Children, pregnant women and women who are trying to get pregnant should not eat shark, swordfish or marlin, which contain more mercury than other types of fish: the developing brain seems to be especially vulnerable to certain chemicals. Other adults should not eat more than one portion of shark, swordfish or marlin per week.

Omega-3 and MS

Northern Norway is an exception to the rule that MS becomes more common the further you get from the equator. Indeed, despite a marked decline in the amount of sunlight, the risk of developing MS declines by up to half the further north you go in Norway. MS rates are also lower in, for example, Japan and Alaska than you would expect based on their distance from the equator.[4]

Fish consumption seems to explain this apparent paradox. The Northern Norwegian diet is rich in fatty fish, especially trout and salmon.[3] The traditional diets of people in Japan and Alaska are also rich in fish. In one study, people who ate the most fish were more than a quarter (28 per cent) less likely to develop MS compared with those who did not eat fish.[79]

In addition, people in northern Norway traditionally consume large amounts of cod liver oil.[3] In one study, people who took cod liver oil between the ages of 13 and 18 years were a third (33 per cent) less likely to develop MS in later life. Cod liver oil did not seem to protect against MS in younger children or adults. This finding is in line with suggestions that adolescents are especially susceptible to the risk factors that lead to MS in later life.[79]

PUFAs or vitamin D?

Originally, researchers thought that omega-3 PUFAs probably accounted for the benefits of fatty fish on MS. Now, however, most researchers believe that vitamin D is responsible. Indeed, the diet in Northern Norway commonly contains about 4,000 IU of vitamin D – that's 10 to 20 times the usual recommended intake.[3] (Because of the risk of side effects discussed below, you should not take this high a dose without first seeking medical advice.) Indeed, in the study of teenagers who received cod liver oil, a vitamin D intake of 600 to 800 IU daily almost halved (54 per cent reduction) their risk of MS.[79]

While vitamin D almost certainly makes an important contribution to the benefits of fish, it is perhaps too soon to write off omega-3 PUFAs and a related group of fatty acids called omega-6 PUFAs. Consider, for example, the benefits listed below.

- Some evidence, albeit from small studies, suggests that a diet rich in omega-3 and omega-6 PUFAs and relatively low in saturated fat may have a mild disease-modifying effect in MS.[19]
- Scandinavian cuisine typically uses canola (also called rapeseed) oil, which contains much higher levels of omega-3 PUFAs than olive oil.[16] Canola oil also contains less saturated fat than olive oil and is rich in vitamin E. You could think about using canola oil in cooking.
- Cold water fish, such as salmon, tuna and sardines, tend to be rich in a type of omega-3 PUFA called docosahexaenoic acid (DHA),[16] which seems to reduce inflammation in the brain.[16]

On the other hand, when scientists reviewed the data, they found that a low-fat diet with fish oil supplementation probably did not reduce relapse, disability or MRI lesions, or improve fatigue or quality of life.[80] Likewise, NICE concluded that 'there is no evidence' that omega-3 and omega-6 PUFAs influence relapse frequency or MS progression. NICE says that the MS team should not offer omega-3 and omega-6 PUFAs *to treat* MS (my italics). Nevertheless, I feel that further studies are probably needed before researchers can draw definitive conclusions.

Despite the mixed evidence of a specific benefit on MS, given the other advantages of eating fish, it seems prudent to eat two portions of fish a week, one of which should be oily fish. Increasing your PUFA intake seems to be beneficial in so many ways that even if it turns out it has no effect on MS, your health generally may well improve.

Vitamin D supplements

As we have seen, exposure to sunlight and eating fatty fish seem to reduce the risk of MS, both of which underscore the importance of vitamin D. There are five forms of vitamin D, of which vitamin D_2 (also called ergocalciferol) and vitamin D_3 (cholecalciferol) are the most important for human health.

The amount of vitamin D in your body depends on the combination of three sources: food, sunlight and supplements or fortification. Sunlight is the main source of vitamin D in the UK, and oily fish is the only important source in the food that most of us eat.[26]

The UK government's Scientific Advisory Committee on Nutrition recommends that everyone in the general UK population aged 4 years and above should get 10 micrograms per day (400 IU per day) of vitamin D throughout the year. This 'Reference Nutrient Intake' aims to ensure that the vitamin D status of 39 in every 40 people (97.5 per cent) is sufficient to protect musculoskeletal health against rickets, osteomalacia and falls, and maintain muscle strength and function.

Vitamin D may also have numerous other non-musculoskeletal health benefits (on reproductive health, heart disease, diabetes, cancer, asthma and MS, for example).[26-28] We also know that low levels of vitamin D increase the risk of experiencing depression,[81] which is common among people with MS.

The Scientific Advisory Committee on Nutrition felt, however, that there was 'insufficient' evidence about these outcomes to inform the Reference Nutrient Intake, so the ideal intake may be higher if further studies confirm these additional benefits. Nevertheless, even based on the current recommendations, about 30 to 40 per cent of the population have low levels of vitamin D in their blood, increasing their risk of bone disease, in winter, compared with 2 to 13 per cent in summer.

Vitamin D and relapse rates

So, would taking vitamin D supplements help people with MS specifically rather than only protecting their bones and perhaps bolstering their health more generally? The evidence is currently mixed. Some studies have failed to find any benefit on relapse or progression. Other studies, however, hint that there may be a benefit.

One study, for example, measured vitamin D levels in 145 people with RRMS over about 28 months, most of whom were taking drugs to modulate the immune system. About half (48 per cent) of the patients experienced at least one relapse. Each 10 nmol/l (the level in the blood) increase in vitamin D seemed to reduce the risk of a relapse by 12 per cent. The benefit was apparent in the winter (14 per cent reduction) and summer (9 per cent reduction) and across a wide range of patients, including smokers, people with darker skin, those who suffered infections, those able to exercise more and so on. The benefit even persisted after excluding people who were deficient in vitamin D. People with MS taking drugs that influenced the immune system and those on other treatments also benefited.[82]

All these figures may be a little difficult to follow, but the 'take home message' is that in this study, which came from Tasmania, people with low exposure to sunlight showed a benefit from increased vitamin D. The same probably applies to less sunny climates. The average vitamin D levels were 41 nmol/l in the winter and 75 nmol/ in the summer – a 34 nmol/ difference. The authors estimate that an increase of 50 nmol/l in vitamin D levels could halve the risk of relapse, which is similar to the effect produced by many drugs.[82] (Note, though, that vitamin D is not a substitute for conventional treatments. It 'supplements' your usual treatment.)

Although very high levels can cause calcium deposits in the lungs, kidney, heart and blood vessels,[3] vitamin D is generally safe and, as it has numerous other benefits, you should ensure that you get enough – whatever the effects on MS. NICE currently recommends, however, that the MS team should not suggest vitamin D solely for treating MS, so if you want to take more than what is suggested in the official recommendations, speak to your MS team.

Salt

Some preliminary evidence suggests that a salt-rich diet may contribute to autoimmune responses in the CNS. For example, in experimental animals, a disease similar to MS was more aggressive in mice fed a high-sodium diet. In human, sodium seems to be linked to increased MS activity both in terms of symptoms and on MRI.[18]

Further studies are needed. In the meantime, however, sticking to the recommended salt intake seems sensible. High-salt diets are also, for example, a leading cause of hypertension (dangerously raised blood pressure) and, therefore, stroke.

The NHS recommends that adults should eat no more than 6 g of salt (2.4 g of sodium) a day – that's about one teaspoon. You soon know that crisps and peanuts are salty. However, many foods contain 'hidden salt': your taste buds will not set alarm bells ringing. For example, manufacturers add surprisingly large amounts of salt to some soups, bread, biscuits, processed meat (including ham and salami), cheese, stock cubes and even ice cream.[83, 84] Indeed, salt added to processed foods accounts for approximately 80 per cent of our total salt intake,[85] so:

- read the label and avoid high-salt foods, which contain more than 1.5 g of salt (0.6 g of sodium) per 100 g. Low-salt foods contain 0.3 g of salt (0.1 g of sodium) or less per 100 g;
- avoid foods – such as smoked meat and fish – that are high in salt;
- add as little salt as you can during baking and cooking;
- banish the salt cellar from the table;

- ask restaurants and take-aways for 'no salt';
- look for low-salt ketchup, pickles, mustard, yeast extract, stock cubes and so on;
- avoid foods that include a chemical name that includes sodium, such as disodium phosphate, monosodium glutamate or sodium nitrate.[86]

If your food seems bland, you could, for example, attend a culinary evening class or work through a range of cook books to increase the amount and variety of spices and herbs you use.

8

Complementary and alternative medicines

Despite using some of the most scientifically advanced drugs, between 1 in 3 (33 per cent) and 4 in 5 (80 per cent) people with MS use CAMs.[80] There's no doubt that many people feel that they benefit from CAMs. And there is some scientific support for certain CAMs in people with MS. Furthermore, it is all too easy to feel disempowered when you face MS, and that you can do little to improve your prospects. CAMs help restore your sense of control over the MS and your life more generally. Nevertheless, as I've stressed several times, CAMs support conventional therapies – they are not replacements.

Some alternative practitioners, however, suggest stopping conventional therapy and using their approach to 'cure' MS, often based on a couple of spectacular 'remissions'. The overwhelming majority of alternative practitioners are well-meaning, kind, honest people who firmly believe that their therapy works. A few are frauds, charlatans and confidence tricksters. (Mind you, some healthcare professionals are far from perfect.) The best advice is to never believe claims that anyone can cure MS when conventional medicine cannot, never stop any conventional treatment or even reduce the dose unless your GP or MS team advises you to and be cautious if a CAM practitioner highlights only one or two remarkable improvements. If it sounds too good to be true, it probably is.

Given the large number of CAMs, it is important to take advice from your MS team or patient group and to read up on the approach you want to try. It is worth making the effort: the following examples illustrate that CAMs can help as part of a holistic approach to living with MS. There are, however, no guarantees. You will invest time, energy, emotion – and often money – in some CAMs. Yet the MS will probably still progress – as we've mentioned several times, there are no cures for MS and even the most effective drugs reduce rather than prevent relapses and progression. Nevertheless, for many people, CAMs help make living with MS easier, improve quality of life and lessen the emotional and psychological impact.

Types of CAM

You can choose from numerous CAMs, from acupuncture to zootherapy – using animals as a treatment. In some cases, for example, animals offer companionship; the care can help create a purpose in life and evoke pleasant memories, which help 'distract' people from their difficulties. And many people talk to their pets. Indeed, some people speak more openly to their pet than their spouse, probably because animals are, obviously, non-judgemental, which helps get problems off the owner's chest.

In addition, walking the dog may help prevent a person with MS from becoming housebound, offer a sense of security and help exercise. Throwing an object for a dog to retrieve helps enhance coordination, builds upper body muscle strength and improves flexibility. Riding a horse improves posture, strength, balance and mobility in people with MS, cerebral palsy, spina bifida, autism and so on. Even a fish tank in a dentist's waiting room is enough to reduce anxiety.[87]

Different approaches, common aims

Mind–body therapies – such as meditation, yoga, visualization, relaxation, hypnosis and biofeedback – differ in approach, but they share an ability to enhance the mind's ability to improve physical and psychological well-being.[57]

Broadly, however, CAMs broadly fall into five groups.[88]

- **Biologically based therapies**, such as diets, vitamins, herbalism and aromatherapy.
- **Energy fields** Some CAM therapists believe that energy fields surround and penetrate the body. They believe that they can manipulate these energy fields using, for example, traditional acupuncture, Reiki and reflexology.
- **Manipulative and body-based CAMs** such as chiropractic, osteopathy, shiatsu, massage and the Alexander technique, which depend on manipulating or moving parts of the body.

It is especially important to be careful and ask your team for advice with manipulative CAMs if the MS or another disease has affected your joints, muscles or bones.

- **Enhancing the mind's ability to influence the body**, using, for example, hypnosis, visualization and spiritual healing. Some approaches – such as shamanic healing or counselling – are predominantly psychological. Nevertheless, by addressing the psychological burden imposed by MS, people often feel better physically.
- **Complete systems**, which include homeopathy, Ayurveda and Traditional Chinese Medicine.

Some CAMs fit into more than one group. During shiatsu, healers apply rhythmic pressure to parts of the body that, they believe, are important for the flow of the 'life force' or qi, so shiatsu is a manipulative and energy field therapy. In addition, healers often take elements from more than one approach to meet their clients' individual needs. Naturopathy combines diet with, for example, herbalism, acupuncture and counselling.[88] This can make it difficult to find out which elements make the difference or whether they all help by tackling different issues faced by the person with MS.

A blurred boundary

It is sometimes hard to see the boundary between mainstream therapy and CAMs. Ayurvedic medicine is mainstream in India, but a CAM in the UK.[88] It is also sometimes hard to see the boundary between alternative and complementary therapies. Broadly, however, alternative therapies *replace* conventional treatments. Sometimes the person's intent makes the difference. Some people will use a CAM alongside the conventional treatment. Someone else will use the same CAM instead of the approach recommended by their doctor. At the risk of labouring the point, the suggestions below are complementary: they do not replace conventional medicine. And always check with your MS team before starting a CAM.

Cynics point to the lack of evidence supporting many CAMs. Certainly, few CAMs undergo the same rigorous testing as modern medicines for MS, but clinical trials are very expensive and pharmaceutical companies fund most trials, so the lack of studies of CAMs is not surprising. In addition, the signs and symptoms of MS wax and wane over time.[89] This makes teasing out whether the improvement is due to the treatment – conventional or CAM – or the natural variation in the course of MS can be difficult. Nevertheless, no evidence of effectiveness is not necessarily the same as evidence of no effect.

The placebo response

In other cases, cynics ascribe CAMs' benefits to the placebo effect. Indeed, the 'placebo response' – the term derives from the Latin phrase for 'I shall please' – contributes to the effectiveness of every conventional drug you take, every CAM or psychotherapy you try, every lifestyle change you make.

The placebo response can be remarkably potent. A surgeon operating near the front line during the Korean War began suffering severe abdominal pain, which he knew indicated acute appendicitis. As incoming wounded personnel needed his help, he asked the nurse to give him a morphine injection. The pain eased and he kept working. With the crisis over, the doctor underwent surgery to remove his appendix.[90]

After returning to duty, the doctor was looking through the operating room records and found that 'since he appeared distressed', the nurse had injected inactive saline and not morphine.[90] (She probably wanted to avoid the mental fogging that morphine can cause.) In other words, a simple salt solution used to mix injectable drugs alleviated the severe pain of acute appendicitis. Critically,

The mind really can affect the body

As the surgeon's experience shows, the mind really can affect the body. Indeed, healers recognized millennia ago that the mind can produce dramatic physical effects and there are countless examples of this. More recently, some people who witnessed the torture and horrors of the Cambodian killing fields reported fuzzy visions or even blindness, yet doctors could find nothing medically wrong with their eyes.[91] On the other hand, some people seem able to postpone their death until after an important event. For example, according to the *New York Times*, the city's death rate in the first week of the new millennium rose by more than half (50.8 per cent) compared with the final week of 1999.

however, the surgeon *expected* the nurse to follow his instructions. He *expected* to receive a powerful painkiller. This expectation invoked the placebo response – his mind and body reacted as if he had received the morphine. For instance, the brain probably released natural painkillers called endorphins.

How placebos work

We are now beginning to understand how certain placebos work. For example, placebos can increase levels of the body's natural painkillers and counter anxiety. The mind and the immune system are also intimately intertwined.

In the early twentieth century, the Russian scientist Ivan Pavlov rang a bell when he fed a dog. Faced with food, the dog salivated. Over time, the dog salivated when Pavlov rang the bell, whether or not he also offered food. Pavlov called this a 'conditioned reflex'.

In the late 1970s, the American scientists Robert Ader and Nicholas Cohen fed rats a mixture of water, saccharine and a drug called cyclophosphamide, which suppresses the immune system. When they stopped cyclophosphamide, but continued the water and saccharine, you might expect the rats' immune systems to have recovered. However, the rats' immune responses remained impaired and they continued to die. In other words, the rats' impaired immune systems became 'conditioned' to the sweet taste of the saccharine.[92]

Since then, scientists have uncovered numerous links that allow the nervous and immune systems to communicate. For example, lymphocytes – a type of white blood cell – produce small message-carrying proteins identical to some of those in the brain. In addition, nerves hard-wire connections between the thymus gland, spleen, lymph nodes and bone marrow, all of which are important parts of the immune system. In 1980, Ader called the study of these connections 'psychoneuroimmunology'.

Such findings help us understand why stress can undermine the immune response and, for example, contribute to triggering a relapse of MS. For example, natural killer cells, another type of white blood cell, attack and destroy infected or cancerous cells. One study of students found that the activity of the natural killer cells declined around the time of their examinations. Another study infected students experimentally with influenza virus. Stressed-out students suffered worse flu symptoms and produced more mucus than their less worried counterparts.[93]

Indeed, placebos contribute to the benefits of conventional medicine. For example, the placebo response may account for up to three-quarters (68 per cent to about 75 per cent) of the benefits offered by antidepressants and up to three-fifths (62 per cent) of the effect of a treatment for peripheral neuropathy (page 33). Sham surgical procedures also have a powerful placebo effect. Indeed, the placebo response can affect the immune system. Some neurologists believe that the placebo effect might account for the improvements seen with some CAMs and less well-established treatments for MS.[89]

Consultation quality

We expect doctors, nurses and CAM practitioners to help. Those doctors and MS teams who raise our expectations and increase our optimism, who are enthusiastic about the treatment, confident, authoritative, empathic, charismatic and warm, seem to bolster the placebo effect and enhance the treatment's intrinsic activity.[90, 91] On the other side of the relationship, a person's desire to believe, 'obey' and please the doctor tends to enhance the placebo response. Not surprisingly, hostility reduces a drug's efficacy,[90, 91] partly by countering the placebo and partly by making poor adherence (page 50) more likely.

You will almost certainly get a 'better quality' and longer consultation with a CAM practitioner than with the average pressurized GP or MS team member. The CAM therapist will ask detailed questions about your medical history, diet, lifestyle, sleeping patterns, likes and dislikes, and so on. This offers you the opportunity to talk to a sympathetic person at greater length than in a conventional consultation about yourself, your fears and concerns, and the practical issues you face living with MS. Not surprisingly, some people find the CAM consultation therapeutic,[88] which can bolster the placebo response of any treatment. Indeed, the quality of your consultation with doctors and nurses also influences the placebo response to conventional medicines.

Do not dismiss these benefits. If you feel better, if life becomes a little easier, it is perhaps less important how you get there. Nevertheless, there is scientific evidence that certain CAMs can help some people with MS.

MS and miracles

Today, headlines regularly proclaim that a new treatment is a 'miracle', often based more on public relations hype than scientific evidence. Yet 'real' – in other words, medically inexplicable – miracles undoubtedly occur.

At the time of writing, the International Medical Committee of Lourdes has recognized 69 miracles among pilgrims to the shrine in south-west France. The committee recognizes miracles only if current science cannot explain the recovery and such recognition is rare. The committee approved the 67th miracle in 1999: an 'inexplicable' improvement in a middle-aged Frenchman with MS. More secular people would suggest a dramatic 'placebo' effect that affected his immune function. Those who are religiously minded will regard the improvement as God's grace and, perhaps, the immunological changes as the way the miracle occurred. Whatever the explanation, these cases show that dramatic improvements in MS occasionally occur.

Acupuncture

Acupuncture is one of the best supported CAMs – and one of the longest-established. Archaeologists uncovered sharpened stones that they believe were used for acupuncture dating from 10,000 BC. The first texts about acupuncture are more than 2,000 years old.

Traditional acupuncture is based on a theory that 12 interconnected channels called meridians connect the body's organs and internal systems. According to practitioners of Traditional Chinese Medicine, qi flows along these meridians. Stimulating these channels – such as by inserting a needle – restores the normal balance and flow of qi.[88] Acupressure stimulates the same points using finger pressure rather than a needle.[53] Sometimes therapists will run a small electrical current through the needle – so-called electroacupuncture.

Acupuncture is a well-established treatment for numerous painful conditions. For instance, a paper in the prestigious *Archives of Internal Medicine* considered 31 studies and reported that acupuncture roughly halved the intensity of chronic pain caused by back, neck and shoulder problems, osteoarthritis and headache. Yet, the paper points out, 'there is no accepted mechanism by which [acupuncture] could have persisting effects on chronic pain'.[94]

Other studies suggested that acupuncture may be a promising treatment for people with MS who experience fatigue, spasticity, pain, or problems with their bowel, bladder, gait and balance. Some studies also report that acupuncture improves quality of life for people with MS. For example, 12 sessions of acupuncture over two months alleviated fatigue in 5 of 20 people who did not respond adequately to amantadine.[95] However, further studies are needed to determine just how effective acupuncture is for people with MS.[95] In the meantime, a qualified acupuncturist will help you decide how they may be able to help you.

Aromatherapy

Your sense of smell may not be anywhere near as sensitive as your dog's or cat's, but it is still powerful. Many people find, for example, that a distinctive smell can evoke childhood memories. Smell helps make food appetising. Aromatherapy uses smells to help improve well-being and quality of life as well as tackling specific problems. For example, some people find that aromatherapy alleviates depression, stress and tiredness. Lavender, for instance, may help alleviate muscle tension and anxiety, and improve sleep. Sweet orange can reduce anxiety.[96] Aromatherapy books are packed with other conditions and problems that this CAM may alleviate.

Aromatherapy uses oils containing concentrated essences taken from flowers, fruit, seeds, leaves, root or bark. There are more than 400 essential oils, some of which are blends. You can use these essential oils in various ways, depending on your problem. You can, for example:

- burn the essential oil or use a diffuser: this can help you meditate or relax (page 94);
- use essential oils in massage, compresses or baths – this might be one way to unwind if you are having difficulty sleeping (page 61);
- apply the oil to acupuncture points or as embrocation – a lotion that alleviates muscle or joint pain.[53]

As ever, check first with your MS team and make sure your

aromatherapist knows that you have MS and what your particular problems are. Some oils, for example, can irritate sensitive skin. It is best to consult a qualified aromatherapist. Massage of some muscles or joints affected by MS may be counterproductive. Always check if you experience spasms, contractures and so on before using any form of manipulation.

Herbal treatment

Plants provide an invaluable source of conventional drugs. In 1763, the English chaplain Edward Stone found that willow bark alleviated ague, a fever caused by malaria that was then rife in parts of England. Aspirin is a chemically modified, less toxic version of the active ingredient in willow bark. Morphine – which remains a mainstay of pain management – comes from a type of poppy. Nabiximols (page 76) is derived from cannabis.

These drugs contain one or two chemicals isolated from the plant. In contrast, herbalists use the whole plant or part of a plant – the root, leaf and so on – rather than one or two chemicals. Herbalists believe that various chemicals in a plant act together to increase effectiveness – so-called synergy. Some components work together to reduce the risk of side effects, which herbalists call buffering. Using several plants together, according to herbalists, further increases activity and buffering.[88]

Herbal treatments are popular. UK studies suggest that between 13 per cent and 44 per cent of adults use herbal remedies[97] and they can help various problems associated with MS. For example, taking *Ginkgo biloba* (240 mg a day for four weeks) was found in one study to reduce fatigue in people with MS compared with placebo.[80]

People with MS may also use herbal treatments to cope with particular issues. The Ancient Egyptians, Greeks and Romans used camomile to alleviate conditions as diverse as colds, sore throats, abscesses, eczema, anxiety and insomnia. Camomile tea contains a chemical called apigenin, which scientific studies confirm is a mild sedative and anxiolytic. Herbalists may suggest camomile as an anti-inflammatory, or to boost immunity, alleviate anxiety, treat diarrhoea or facilitate sleep.[98] Valerian is another 'classic' herbal remedy used to improve fatigue, reduce drowsiness and improve sleep,[49] but, like any drug, it is best to use it and the other herbal remedies for only a few weeks while sleep hygiene (page 61) begins to restore a restful night.

Rather than treating yourself using herbs, it is best to consult a qualified medical herbalist and make sure to tell him or her about any disease or ailment or any conventional medicines you are taking. Your GP and MS team needs to know about any herbal remedy you're taking as some herbs can interact with conventional medicines (page 49).

Medical marijuana

Few medicines have been as widely used, for as long, as *Cannabis sativa*. Babylonians probably used cannabis as an incense in their temples in the third millennium BC. Millennia later, in 1842, the army surgeon William O'Shaughnessy introduced cannabis into British medicine inspired by traditional uses of the herb he had seen during his posting to India. The Victorians used cannabis to induce sleep and childbirth as well as to alleviate, among other ailments, muscle spasms, menstrual cramps, rheumatism, tetanus, rabies and epilepsy. As we have seen, nabiximols (page 76), which is derived from cannabis, is effective for moderate to severe spasticity.

Medical marijuana is legal in several parts of the world and numerous websites extol its virtues. The UK government, however, banned the recreational use of cannabis in 1928 and medical use in 1973. Medical marijuana remains illegal in the UK.

Reflexology and massage

Reflexologists massage points on the feet that they believe stimulate another part of the body. Massaging the tip of the big toe, for example, is believed to stimulate the top of the head.[99] One study compared ten 45-minute weekly sessions of foot massage against reflexology.[80] Foot massage and reflexology seemed to reduce pain, disability, spasticity, fatigue and depression. Another study compared 11 weekly sessions that combined reflexology and calf massage with calf massage alone. Reflexology seemed to reduce paraesthesia, urinary symptoms and spasticity more than calf massage alone. Paraesthesia seemed to show an especially marked improvement.[80]

Even if you do not accept the idea of a link between areas of your feet and certain other parts of the body, many people find a foot massage helps them relax and improves their well-being. Make sure you consult an experienced masseur and check with the MS team first. Inappropriate pressure, for example, can cause pain, and joint or tissue manipulation may not be suitable for everyone.

Biofeedback

Biofeedback allows you to influence parts of your body that usually work without conscious control, such as heartbeat, blood pressure, respiration rate and muscle tension. Biofeedback machines and software typically make a sound or show a display that varies according to the activity of, for example, your heartbeat. By listening to the sounds or watching the display, you train yourself to regulate the signals and, in turn, exert some control over your body's unconscious functions. Biofeedback helps several symptoms that can occur in MS, including bladder incontinence, anxiety, pain and constipation.[57] As we have seen, biofeedback can also help with balance and motor difficulties (page 71).

Tai chi

Tai chi (tai chi chuan) is a 'soft' or 'internal' martial art that combines deep breathing, meditation and relaxation with sequences (called forms) of slow, gentle movements that enhance fitness, strength and flexibility. As such, tai chi is often suitable (after checking with your doctor) for people with MS and other long-term diseases.

Tai chi's slow, gentle movements improve strength, balance, posture, concentration, relaxation and breath control, so it can help to prevent falls and improve how well your heart and lungs work.[100] Exercise can improve strength, fitness, mobility, mood, fatigue and quality of life for people with MS.[101] In addition to improving strength and flexibility, tai chi offers a form of meditation (or mindfulness) and helps you become more aware of your body.[101]

In one study, balance in women with MS improved after a 12-week course of tai chi sessions twice a week.[51] During another study, people with MS participated in tai chi sessions twice a week for six months. Each session lasted 90 minutes. Another group received usual treatment. Balance, coordination, depression and satisfaction with life all improved in the people who took part in tai chi. Fatigue worsened in the 'usual care' group, but did not get any worse in the tai chi group.[101]

Tai chi may look undemanding until you try it. You can learn the tai chi short form in about 12 lessons, although tai chi takes many years to fully master. Speeded up, tai chi can offer effective self-defence – indeed, *chuan* means 'fist'. Speed up a raising hand and you may deflect a blow to the head. Speeded up, a descending hand can deflect a kick. Qi gong also combines deep breathing, meditation, relaxation and movements. However, the movements are more internally focused on the 'flow of energy' around the body than they are in tai chi.

Guided imagery

The mind and body are intimately intertwined. Sports people know this: they improve their performance by imagining the goal going in, how they'll win the race or make the touchdown.

Essentially, the images 'serve as a bridge between the mind and body'. Guided imagery and visualization use your imagination to change your body, mind and emotions and help you cope with MS.[53] You might visualize a soothing feeling around a sore part of your body, for example. You might visualize a 'safe place' (it can be a made-up place or a favourite haunt) when you are uncomfortable, stressed or anxious, such as before an injection. The more you call the image to mind, the stronger the image becomes and the greater the benefit will be.

Guided imagery takes visualization a step further. During guided imagery you use imagery, metaphor, story-telling, fantasy exploration and game-playing. You can do this on your own – several books can teach you the principles – although many people find it helps to have a therapist guide the internal journey. During guided imagery, you will imagine yourself performing a task ideally including the accompanying sensations. Some people find that guided imagery and visualization can improve energy, sleep and digestion, and counter stress, anxiety, pain and fatigue. Guided imagery and visualization may boost the immune system and improve emotional control.[53] However, guided imagery may not be suitable for people with MS who develop marked cognitive impairment.[57]

Hypnosis

For centuries, conventional doctors dismissed hypnotism as a stage trick, its benefits confined to weak-willed, gullible people. Some doctors even suggested that subjects 'faked' responses to please their hypnotist.

Yet in the early nineteenth century, there were no effective anaesthetics. Patients usually needed to be drunk and tied down before the surgeon operated. Then, in 1829, the French doctor Pierre-Jean Chapelain used hypnosis as an anaesthetic during a mastectomy for breast cancer. In the 1840s, James Esdaile, a Scottish surgeon working near Calcutta, removed a scrotal tumour using hypnosis as anaesthesia.[36, 102] It is hard to believe someone would endure the pain of a mastectomy or scrotal operation just to please the surgeon. Today, we have powerful painkillers and anaesthetics, but these examples show the power of hypnotism.

Doctors do not fully understand how hypnotism works. Essentially, however, hypnosis is focused attention and concentration.[36, 103] Some hypnotists describe the process as similar to being 'so lost in a book or movie that it is easy to lose track of what is going on around you'.[36] Dissociation (you move competing stimuli to the edge of your awareness) and suggestibility (you go along with the hypnotist's suggestion) probably contribute.

Hypnotism and MS

While the mechanism may be unclear, many people with MS find that hypnotism alleviates some symptoms, including pain, fatigue, distress, nausea and vomiting. Hypnosis can help change harmful habits, such as abusing alcohol, comfort eating or smoking. Hypnotists can provide coping strategies, such as replacing pain with a numb or cool sensation.[103] In one study, 87 per cent of people with MS who used self-hypnosis reported at least a 30 per cent decrease in pain intensity.[47]

Hypnosis is safe. You won't lose control: a hypnotist cannot make you do or say anything he or she wants. You will be able to come 'out' of hypnosis whenever you want.[36] Some people also find that self-hypnosis helps. Numerous DVDs, CDs and books can help you create the 'focused attention' that underpins hypnosis.

Yoga

Yoga brings millions of people – from all religious backgrounds – inner peace, relief from stress and improved health. Yoga aims to harmonize consciousness, mind, energy and body. (The Indian root of the word yoga means 'to unite'.)

Essentially, yoga focuses on achieving controlled, slow, deep breaths, while the poses (asanas) increase fitness, strength and flexibility. As a result, yoga helps maintain suppleness of both body and mind. Some poses require considerable concentration.

Yoga and mindfulness seem to improve fatigue in people with MS.[57] Over eight weeks, yoga and aquatic exercise in addition to standard treatments seemed to reduce the risk of developing fatigue, depression and paraesthesia in people with MS compared with those who did not exercise. Indeed, people who took part in yoga or the aquatic exercise were 35 times less likely to develop moderate or severe depression than those who did not exercise.[48]

If you have musculoskeletal problems, you can ask the yoga teacher whether cushions, blocks, straps and so on can help you hold the asasna.[57] You might want to avoid bikram yoga, which is performed in a heated room and can therefore exacerbate symptoms of MS (page 15). You could try to find a yoga teacher who is experienced teaching people with disabilities.[57]

Using CAMs safely

If you want to try a CAM, check with your MS team first and consult a registered practitioner, such as one recognized by the General Regulatory Council for Complementary Therapies or the Complementary and Natural Healthcare Council. Read up on the approach you are planning to use – this chapter only briefly considers a few examples – and make sure you understand the risks and benefits. You should tell the CAM practitioner that you have MS and which treatments you are taking. Ideally, the CAM practitioner should be experienced in treating people with MS. You could ask your team or other people with MS if they know of a practitioner.

Watch for side effects. For example, some alternative healers believe that CAMs drive out toxins that have accumulated in your body. Some of these, some healers believe, may be contributing to your MS or undermining your immune system. They say that this toxic 'tsunami' can produce a detox 'crisis', characterized by, for example, headaches, fatigue and abdominal discomfort. In some cases, the healer and person undergoing detox can dismiss adverse events as such a crisis, so you need to be careful if you experience any unexpected symptoms: they may be sign of a relapse, a side effect of the CAM or conventional therapy – or something else.

Keep an eye on whether or not the CAM is working. You could keep a diary to track the improvement over three to four months and then speak to the CAM and MS team if you feel it is not working. It might be time to consider another approach. On the other hand, if CAM works well, do not reduce the dose of, or stop taking, any of the conventional drugs without speaking to your GP or MS team first.

As already stressed, never believe claims that a particular CAM can cure MS, or follow advice to stop a conventional therapy or eat a highly restricted diet that goes against the advice of the dietitian on your MS team. The CAM practitioner is often acting with the best of intentions. However, your best chance of alleviating symptoms and living a full live despite MS comes from using CAMs alongside conventional treatments.

A final word

Over the last few years, scientists have made remarkable advances in our understanding of the causes of MS. The MS team can offer a growing and increasingly effective range of treatments that reduce the risk of relapses and slow the decline into disability. Some of these advances, stem cells for example, could potentially revolutionize management, although it's still early days. Some CAMs are beginning to reach the medical mainstream, as studies confirm their worth. Despite these remarkable advances, however, MS remains stubbornly enigmatic and incurable. Nevertheless, we have seen throughout this book that you and your carer can work with your MS team to live full and rich lives. I wish you well.

Useful addresses

British Association for Behavioural and Cognitive Psychotherapies
Imperial House
Hornby Street
Bury
Lancashire BL9 5BN
Tel.: 0161 705 4304
Website: www.babcp.com

British Dietetic Association
5th Floor, Charles House,
148/9 Great Charles Street Queensway
Birmingham B3 3HT
Tel.: 0121 200 8080
Website: www.bda.uk.com

Carers Direct
Tel.: 0300 123 1053 (helpline)
Website: www.nhs.uk/carersdirect

Complementary and Natural Healthcare Council
46–48 Smithfield
London E1W 1AW
Tel.: 020 3668 0406
Website: www.cnhc.org.uk

Federation of Holistic Therapists
18 Shakespeare Business Centre
Hathaway Close
Eastleigh SO50 4SR
Tel.: 023 8062 4350
Website: www.fht.org.uk

General Regulatory Council for Complementary Therapies
Box 437, Office 6
Slington House
Rankine Road
Basingstoke RG24 8PH
Tel.: 0870 3144031
Website: www.grcct.org

Health and Care Professions Council
Park House
184 Kennington Park Road
London SE11 4BU
Tel.: 0300 500 6184
Website: www.hpc-uk.org

Institute for Complementary and Natural Medicine (and British Register of Complementary Practitioners)
Can-Mezzanine
32–36 Loman Street
London SE1 0EH
Tel.: 020 7922 7980
Website: www.icnm.org.uk

MS Research and Relief Fund
Benmar House
Choppington Road
Stobhill
Morpeth
Northumberland NE61 2HX
Tel.: 01670 505829
Website: www.ms-researchandrelief.org

MS Research Treatment and Education
MS Research
The Vassall Centre
Gill Avenue
Fishponds
Bristol BS16 2QQ
Tel.: 0117 958 6986
Website: www.ms-research.org.uk/index.php

MS Society
MS National Centre
372 Edgware Road
London NW2 6ND
Tel.: 0808 800 8000 (helpline)
Website: www.mssociety.org.uk

Multiple Sclerosis Trust
Spirella Building
Bridge Road
Letchworth Garden City
Hertfordshire SG6 4ET
Tel.: 0800 032 3839
Website: www.mstrust.org.uk

Multiple Sclerosis International Federation
3rd Floor
Skyline House
200 Union Street
London SE1 0LX
Tel: 020 7620 1911
Website: www.msif.org

MS-Ireland
80 Northumberland Road
Dublin 4
Tel.: +44 850 233233 (helpline)
Website: www.ms-society.ie
MS-UK
Tel.: 0800 783 0518 (helpline)
Website: www.ms-uk.org

National Multiple Sclerosis Society (US site)
Tel.: 00 1 880 344 4867
Website: www.nationalmssociety.org

National Institute of Medical Herbalists
Clover House
James Court
South Street
Exeter EX1 1EE
Tel.: 01392 426022
Website: www.nimh.org.uk

NHS Smokefree
Tel.: 0300 123 1044 (national helpline)
Website: www.nhs.uk/smokefree

Tai Chi Union for Great Britain
Peter Ballam
Secretary
5 Corunna Drive
Horsham
West Sussex RH13 5HG
Website: www.taichiunion.com

References

1   Quoted in de Vries, J. (1985) *Multiple Sclerosis.* Edinburgh: Mainstream Publishing.

2   Feinstein, A., Freeman, J. and Lo, A. C. (2015) 'Treatment of progressive multiple sclerosis: What works, what does not, and what is needed', *The Lancet Neurology*, 14: 194–207.

3   Amor, S. and Van Noort, H. (2012) *Multiple Sclerosis: The facts.* Oxford: Oxford University Press.

4   Greenberg, B. M. (2016) 'Vitamin D during pregnancy and multiple sclerosis: An evolving association', *JAMA Neurology*, 73(5): 498–9 (DOI:10.1001/jamaneurol.2016.0018).

5   Mackenzie, I. S., Morant, S. V., Bloomfield, G. A., MacDonald, T. M. and O'Riordan, J. (2014) 'Incidence and prevalence of multiple sclerosis in the UK 1990–2010: A descriptive study in the General Practice Research Database', *The Journal of Neurology, Neurosurgery and Psychiatry*, 85: 76–84.

6   Scolding, N. and Wilkins, A. (2012) *Multiple Sclerosis.* Oxford: Oxford University Press.

7   Albor, C., du Sautoy, T., Kali Vanan, N., Turner, B. P., Boomla, K. and Schmierer, K. (2016) 'Ethnicity and prevalence of multiple sclerosis in east London'. *Multiple Sclerosis Journal*, 17 March, pii (DOI: 10.1177/1352458516638746).

8   Greener. M. (2012) 'Rehabilitation for multiple sclerosis: Bridging the gaps', *Progress in Neurology and Psychiatry*, 16: 7–8.

9   Kumar, D. R., Aslinia, F., Yale, S. H. and Mazza, J. J. (2011) 'Jean-Martin Charcot: The father of neurology', *Clinical Medicine and Research*, 9: 46–9.

10 Grytten, N., Aarseth, J. H., Lunde, H. M. B and Myhr, K. M. (2016) 'A 60-year follow-up of the incidence and prevalence of multiple sclerosis in Hordaland County, Western Norway', *The Journal of Neurology, Neurosurgery and Psychiatry*, 87: 100–5.

11 Holick, M. F. (2007) 'Vitamin D deficiency', *New England Journal of Medicine*, 357: 266–81.

12 Siegel, A. and Sapru, H. (2010) *Essential Neuroscience* (2nd edn). Baltimore, MD: Lippincott Williams & Wilkins.

13 Benz, C. and Reynolds, R. (2004) *Coping with Multiple Sclerosis.* London: Vermillion.

14 Burdett, T. C. and Freeman, M. R. (2014) 'Astrocytes eyeball axonal mitochondria', *Science*, 345: 385–6.

15 Hood, B. (2014) *The Domesticated Brain.* London: Pelican.

16 Stetka, B. (2016) 'In search of the optimal brain diet', *Scientific American Mind*, 27: 26–33.

17 Greener, M. (2015) 'Don't underestimate glial cells', *Progress in Neurology and Psychiatry*, 19: 5–8.

18 Garg, N. and Smith, T. W. (2015) 'An update on immunopathogenesis, diagnosis, and treatment of multiple sclerosis', *Brain and Behavior*, 5(9): e00362.

19 Halper, J. and Holland, N. (2010) *Comprehensive Nursing Care in Multiple Sclerosis* (3rd edn). New York: Springer.

20 Belbasis, L., Bellou, V., Evangelou, E., Ioannidis, J. P. and Tzoulaki, I. (2015) 'Environmental risk factors and multiple sclerosis: An umbrella review of systematic reviews and meta-analyses', *The Lancet Neurology*, 14: 263–73.

21 Monteiro, L., Souza-Machado, A., Menezes, C. and Melo, A. (2011) 'Association between allergies and multiple sclerosis: A systematic review and meta-analysis', *Acta Neurologica Scandinavica*, 123: 1–7.

22 Davidson, P. W., Myers, G. J. and Weiss, B. (2004) 'Mercury exposure and child development outcomes', *Pediatrics*, 113: 1023–9.

23 Annunziato, A. (2008) 'DNA packaging: Nucleosomes and chromatin', *Nature Education*, 1: 26.

24 Hollenbach, J. A. and Oksenberg, J. R. (2015) 'The immunogenetics of multiple sclerosis: A comprehensive review', *The Journal of Autoimmunity*, 64: 13–25.

25 Lewis, D. (1992) 'What was wrong with Tiny Tim?', *The American Journal of Diseases of Children*, 146: 1403–7.

26 NICE (2014) 'Vitamin D: Increasing supplement use among at-risk groups'. Available online at: <www.nice.org.uk/guidance/PH56>.

27 Hou, W., Yan, X. T., Bai, C. M., Zhang, X. W., Hui, L. Y and Yu, X. W. (2016) 'Decreased serum vitamin D levels in early spontaneous pregnancy loss', *European Journal of Clinical Nutrition*, 70: 1004–8.

28 Martineau, A., Cates, C., Urashima, M., Jensen, M., Griffiths, A. P., Nurmatov, U. et al. (2016) 'Vitamin D for the management of asthma', *Cochrane Database of Systematic Reviews*, 9: CD011511.

29 Munger, K. L., Åivo, J., Hongell, K., Soilu-Hänninen, M., Surcel, H. M. and Ascherio, A. (2016) 'Vitamin D status during pregnancy and risk of multiple sclerosis in offspring of women in the Finnish maternity cohort', *JAMA Neurology*, 73: 515–19.

30 Royal College of Obstetricians and Gynaecologists (2014) 'Vitamin D in pregnancy (Scientific Impact Paper No.43)'. Available online at: <www.rcog.org.uk/en/guidelines-research-services/guidelines/sip43/>.

31 Goldberg, P. (1974) 'Multiple sclerosis: Vitamin D and calcium as environmental determinants of prevalence. Part 1: Sunlight, dietary factors and epidemiology', *International Journal of Environmental Studies*, 6: 19–27.

32 Goldberg, P. (1974) 'Multiple sclerosis: Vitamin D and calcium as environmental determinants of prevalence. Part 2: Biochemical and genetic factors', *International Journal of Environmental Studies*, 6: 121–9.

33   Roossinck, M. (2016) *Virus: An illustrated guide to 101 incredible microbes*. Brighton: Ivy Press.

34   Ramanujam, R., Hedström, A., Manouchehrinia, A., Alfredsson, L., Olsson, T., Bottai M. et al. (2015) 'Effect of smoking cessation on multiple sclerosis prognosis', *JAMA Neurology*, 72: 1117–23.

35   Clancy, N., Zwar, N. and Richmond, R. (2014) 'Depression, smoking and smoking cessation: A qualitative study', *Family Practice*, 30: 587–92.

36   Montgomery, G. H., Schnur, J. B. and Kravits, K. (2013) 'Hypnosis for cancer care: Over 200 years young', *CA: A Cancer Journal for Clinicians*, 63: 31–44.

37   Murray, T. J. (2009) 'The history of multiple sclerosis: The changing frame of the disease over the centuries', *The Journal of the Neurological Sciences*, 277: S3–8.

38   Ramírez, B. and Palacio, V. (2013) 'JC virus: A brief review', *World Journal of Neuroscience*, 3: 126–30.

39   Baldwin, K. J. and Hogg, J. P. (2013) 'Progressive multifocal leukoencephalopathy in patients with multiple sclerosis', *Current Opinion in Neurology*, 26: 318–23.

40   Javed, A. and Reder, A. T. (2016) 'Rising JCV-Ab index during natalizumab therapy for MS: Inauspicious for a highly efficacious drug', *Neurology: Neuroimmunology and Neuroinflammation*, 3: e199.

41   Tsivgoulis, G., Katsanos, A. H., Grigoriadis, N., Hadjigeorgiou, G. M., Heliopoulos, I., Papathanasopoulos, P. et al. (2015) 'The effect of disease modifying therapies on disease progression in patients with relapsing–remitting multiple sclerosis: A systematic review and meta-analysis', *PLoS ONE*, 10: e0144538.

42   Ghezzi, A., Grimaldi, L. M. E., Marrosu, M. G., Pozzilli, C., Comi, G., Bertolotto, A. et al. (2011) 'Natalizumab therapy of multiple sclerosis: Recommendations of the Multiple Sclerosis Study Group–Italian Neurological Society', *Neurological Sciences*, 32: 351–8.

43   Costello, K., Kennedy, P. and Scanzillo, J. (2008) 'Recognizing non-adherence in patients with multiple sclerosis and maintaining treatment adherence in the long term', *Medscape Journal of Medicine*, 10: 225.

44   Henderson, L., Yue, Q. Y., Bergquist, C., Gerden, B. and Arlett, P. (2002) 'St John's wort (*Hypericum perforatum*): Drug interactions and clinical outcomes', *British Journal of Clinical Pharmacology*, 54: 349–56.

45   Steinberg, S. C., Faris, R. J., Chang, C. F., Chan, A. and Tankersley, M. A. (2010) 'Impact of adherence to interferons in the treatment of multiple sclerosis', *Clinical Drug Investigation*, 30: 89–100.

46   Ghahari, S. and Forwell, S. J. (2016) 'Social media representation of chronic cerebrospinal venous insufficiency intervention for multiple sclerosis', *International Journal of MS Care*, 18: 49–57.

47   Jensen, M. P., Barber, J., Romano, J. M., Molton, I. R., Raichle, K. A., Osborne, T. L. et al. (2009) 'A comparison of self-hypnosis versus progressive muscle relaxation in patients with multiple sclerosis

and chronic pain', *International Journal of Clinical and Experimental Hypnosis*, 57: 198–221.

48 Razazian, N., Yavari, Z., Farnia, V., Azizi, A., Kordavani, L., Bahmani, D. S. et al. (2016) 'Exercising impacts on fatigue, depression, and paresthesia in female patients with multiple sclerosis', *Medicine and Science in Sports and Exercise*, 48: 796–803.

49 Hammer, M. J., Ercolano, E. A., Wright, F., Dickson, V. V., Chyun, D. and Melkus, G. D. (2015) 'Self-management for adult patients with cancer: An integrative review', *Cancer Nursing*, 38: E10–26.

50 Lockey, S. and Foster, R. (2012) *Sleep: A very short introduction*. Oxford: Oxford University Press.

51 Azimzadeh, E., Hosseini, M. A., Nourozi, K. and Davidson, P. M. (2014) 'Effect of Tai Chi Chuan on balance in women with multiple sclerosis', *Complementary Therapies in Clinical Practice*, 21: 57–60.

52 Diamant, N. E. (2012) 'Functional anatomy and physiology of swallowing and esophageal motility', in J. E. Richter and D. O. Castell (eds), *The Esophagus* (5th edn). Oxford: Wiley-Blackwell, pp. 63–96.

53 Newton, S., Hickey, M. and Marrs, J. (2009) *Mosby's Oncology Nursing Advisor: A comprehensive guide to clinical practice*. St Louis, MO: Mosby.

54 Manouchehrinia, A., Tanasescu, R., Tench, C. R. and Constantinescu, C. S. (2016) 'Mortality in multiple sclerosis: Meta-analysis of standardised mortality ratios', *The Journal of Neurology, Neurosurgery and Psychiatry*, 87: 324–31.

55 Strohecker, J. and Strohecker, N. (eds) (1999) *Natural Healing for Depression*. New York: Perigee.

56 Edwards, V. (2003) *Depression: What you really need to know*. London: Robinson.

57 Senders, A., Wahbeh, H., Spain, R. and Shinto, L. (2012) 'Mind–body medicine for multiple sclerosis: A systematic review', *Autoimmune Diseases*, 2012: 12.

58 Marrie, R. A., Patten, S. B., Tremlett, H., Wolfson, C., Warren, S., Svenson, L. W. et al. (2016) 'Sex differences in comorbidity at diagnosis of multiple sclerosis: A population-based study', *Neurology*, pii: 10.1212/wnl.0000000000002481.

59 Jones, K. H., Jones, P. A., Middleton, R. M., Ford, D. V., Tuite-Dalton, K., Lockhart-Jones, H. et al. (2014) 'Physical disability, anxiety and depression in people with MS: An internet-based survey via the UK MS register', *PLoS ONE*, 9: e104604.

60 Tylee, A. and Gandhi, P. (2005) 'The importance of somatic symptoms in depression in primary care', *Primary Care Companion to the Journal of Clinical Psychiatry*, 7: 167–76.

61 Russell, A. (2009) *The Social Basis of Medicine*. Oxford: Wiley Blackwell.

62 Hoge, E. A., Ivkovic, A. and Fricchione, G. L. (2012) 'Generalized anxiety disorder: Diagnosis and treatment', *British Medical Journal*, 345: e7500.

63 Simpson, R., Booth, J., Lawrence, M., Byrne, S., Mair, F. and Mercer,

S. (2014) 'Mindfulness based interventions in multiple sclerosis – a systematic review', *BMC Neurology*, 14: 1–9.

64 Pizzagalli, D. A., Bogdan, R., Ratner, K. G. and Jahn, A. L. (2007) 'Increased perceived stress is associated with blunted hedonic capacity: Potential implications for depression research', *Behavior Research and Therapy*, 45: 2742–53.

65 Kirsch, I. (2009) *The Emperor's New Drugs: Exploding the antidepressant myth*. London: Bodley Head.

66 Raissi, A., Bulloch, A. G. M., Fiest, K. M., McDonald, K., Jetté, N. and Patten, S. B. (2015) 'Exploration of undertreatment and patterns of treatment of depression in multiple sclerosis', *International Journal of MS Care*, 17: 292–300.

67 Gould J. (2014) 'Mental health: Stressed students reach out for help', *Nature*, 512: 223–4.

68 Jick, S. S., Li, L., Falcone, G. J., Vassilev, Z. P. and Wallander, M. A. (2015) 'Epidemiology of multiple sclerosis: Results from a large observational study in the UK', *The Journal of Neurology*, 262: 2033–41.

69 Hedström, A. K., Mowry, E. M., Gianfrancesco, M. A., Shao, X., Schaefer, C. A., Shen, L. et al. (2016) 'High consumption of coffee is associated with decreased multiple sclerosis risk: Results from two independent studies', *The Journal of Neurology, Neurosurgery and Psychiatry*, 87: 454–60.

70 Dorit, R. (2014) 'The Superorganism revolution', *American Scientist*, 102: 330–3.

71 Perlman, R. (2013) *Evolution and Medicine*. Oxford: Oxford University Press.

72 Stojančević, M., Bojić, G., Salami, H. and Mikov, M. (2013) 'The influence of intestinal tract and probiotics on the fate of orally administered drugs', *Current Issues in Molecular Biology*, 16: 55–68.

73 Zhu, Q., Gao, R., Wu, W. and Qin, H. (2013) 'The role of gut microbiota in the pathogenesis of colorectal cancer', *Tumor Biology*, 34: 1285–300.

74 Le Chatelier, E., Nielsen, T., Qin, J., Prifti, E., Hildebrand, F., Falony, G. et al. (2013) 'Richness of human gut microbiome correlates with metabolic markers', *Nature*, 500: 541–6.

75 Haghikia, A. and Gold, R. (2016) 'Positive effect on multiple sclerosis with treatment of metabolic syndrome', *JAMA Neurology*, 73: 499–501.

76 Jangi, S., Gandhi, R., Cox, L. M., Li, N., von Glehn, F., Yan, R. et al. (2015) 'Alterations of the human gut microbiome in multiple sclerosis', *Nature Communications*, 7: 12015.

77 Chen, J., Chia, N., Kalari, K. R., Yao, J. Z., Novotna, M., Soldan, M. M. et al. (2016) 'Multiple sclerosis patients have a distinct gut microbiota compared to healthy controls', *Scientific Reports*, 6: 28484.

78 Mielcarz, D. W. and Kasper, L. H. (2015) 'The gut microbiome in multiple sclerosis', *Current Treatment Options in Neurology*, 17: 1–10.

79 Cortese, M., Riise, T., Bjørnevik, K., Holmøy, T., Kampman, M. T.,

Magalhaes, S. et al. (2015) 'Timing of use of cod liver oil, a vitamin D source, and multiple sclerosis risk: The EnvIMS study', *Multiple Sclerosis*, 21: 1856–64.

80 Yadav, V., Bever, C., Bowen, J., Bowling, A., Weinstock-Guttman, B., Cameron, M. et al. (2014) 'Summary of evidence-based guideline: Complementary and alternative medicine in multiple sclerosis: Report of the Guideline Development Subcommittee of the American Academy of Neurology', *Neurology*, 82: 1083–92.

81 Sarris, J., Logan, A. C., Akbaraly, T. N., Amminger, G. P., Balanzá-Martínez, V., Freeman, M. P. et al. (2015) 'Nutritional medicine as mainstream in psychiatry', *The Lancet Psychiatry*, 2: 271–4.

82 Simpson, S., Taylor, B., Blizzard, L., Ponsonby, A. L., Pittas, F., Tremlett, H. et al. (2010) 'Higher 25-hydroxyvitamin D is associated with lower relapse risk in multiple sclerosis', *Annals of Neurology*, 68: 193–203.

83 Royal College of Physicians Intercollegiate Stroke Working Party (2012) *National Clinical Guideline for Stroke* (4th edn). London: Royal College of Physicians. Available online at: <www.rcplondon.ac.uk/sites/default/files/national-clinical-guidelines-for-stroke-fourth-edition.pdf>.

84 Lindley, R. (2008) *Stroke: The facts*. Oxford: Oxford University Press.

85 He, F., Pombo-Rodrigues, S. and MacGregor, G. (2014) 'Salt reduction in England from 2003 to 2011: Its relationship to blood pressure, stroke and ischaemic heart disease mortality', *BMJ Open*, 4: e004549.

86 Larkin, M. (1995) *When Someone You Love Has a Stroke*. New York: Dell.

87 Matuszek, S. (2010) 'Animal-facilitated therapy in various patient populations: Systematic literature review', *Holistic Nursing Practice*, 24: 187–203.

88 Russell, A. (2009) *The Social Basis of Medicine*. Chichester: Wiley-Blackwell.

89 Murray, D. and Stoessl, A. J. (2013) 'Mechanisms and therapeutic implications of the placebo effect in neurological and psychiatric conditions', *Pharmacology and Therapeutics*, 140: 306–18.

90 Wall, P. (1993) 'Pain and the placebo response', *Ciba Foundation Symposium*, 174: 187–211; discussion 2–6.

91 Vallance, A. K. (2006) 'Something out of nothing: The placebo effect', *Advances in Psychiatric Treatment*, 12: 287–96.

92 Harrington, A. (2008) *The Cure Within: A history of mind–body medicine*. New York: W. W. Norton.

93 Byrne-Davis, L. and Vedhara, K. (2008) 'Psychoneuroimmunology', *Social and Personality Psychology Compass*, 2: 751–64.

94 Vickers, A. J., Cronin, A. M., Maschino, A. C., Lewith, G., MacPherson, H., Foster, N. E. et al. (2012) 'Acupuncture for chronic pain: Individual patient data meta-analysis', *Archives of Internal Medicine*, 172: 1444–53.

95 Karpatkin, H. I., Napolione, D. and Siminovich-Blok, B. (2014)

'Acupuncture and multiple sclerosis: A review of the evidence', *Evidence-Based Complementary and Alternative Medicine*, 2014: 9.

96 Lehrner, J., Eckersberger, C., Walla, P., Pötsch, G. and Deecke, L. (2000) 'Ambient odor of orange in a dental office reduces anxiety and improves mood in female patients', *Physiology and Behavior*, 71: 83–6.

97 Constable, S., Ham, A. and Pirmohamed, M. (2007) 'Herbal medicines and acute medical emergency admissions to hospital', *British Journal of Clinical Pharmacology*, 63: 247–8.

98 Chang, S.-M. and Chen, C.-H. (2016) 'Effects of an intervention with drinking chamomile tea on sleep quality and depression in sleep disturbed postnatal women: A randomized controlled trial', *The Journal of Advanced Nursing*, 72: 306–15.

99 Rowlands, B. (1997) *The Which? Guide to Complementary Medicine*. London: Which? Books.

100 Chen, Y.-W., Hunt, M. A., Campbell, K. L., Peill, K. and Reid, W. D. (2015) 'The effect of Tai Chi on four chronic conditions – cancer, osteoarthritis, heart failure and chronic obstructive pulmonary disease: A systematic review and meta-analyses'. *British Journal of Sports Medicine*, 50: 397–407.

101 Burschka, J. M., Keune, P. M., Oy, U. H., Oschmann, P. and Kuhn, P. (2014) 'Mindfulness-based interventions in multiple sclerosis: Beneficial effects of Tai Chi on balance, coordination, fatigue and depression', *BMC Neurology*, 14: 165.

102 Bivins, R. (2007) *Alternative Medicine? A history*. Oxford: Oxford University Press.

103 Kravits, K. G. (2015) 'Hypnosis for the management of anticipatory nausea and vomiting', *The Journal of the Advanced Practitioner in Oncology*, 6: 225–9.

Further reading

Amor, S. and Van Noort, H. (2012) *Multiple Sclerosis: The facts*. Oxford: Oxford University Press.

Benz, C. and Reynolds, R. (2004) *Coping with Multiple Sclerosis*. London: Vermillion.

de Vries, J. (1985) *Multiple Sclerosis*. Edinburgh: Mainstream Publishing.

Greener, M. (2015) *Depression and Anxiety: The drug-free way*. London: Sheldon Press.

Greener, M. (2013) *The Holistic Health Handbook*. London: Sheldon Press.

Hood, B. (2014) *The Domesticated Brain*. London: Pelican.

Rawlands, B. (1997) *The Which? Guide to Complementary Medicine*. London: Which? Books

Roossinck, M. (2016) *Virus: An illustrated guide to 101 incredible microbes*. Brighton: Ivy Press.

Scolding, N. and Wilkins, A. (2012) *Multiple Sclerosis*. Oxford: Oxford University Press.

Index